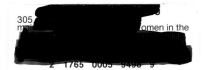

DATE DUE

OCT 2 2 1985		
XXXXXXXXX1988		

Women in the World-System

Women in the World-System
Its Impact on Status and Fertility

by Kathryn B. Ward

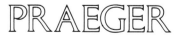

PRAEGER

PRAEGER SPECIAL STUDIES • PRAEGER SCIENTIFIC

New York • Philadelphia • Eastbourne, UK
Toronto • Hong Kong • Tokyo • Sydney

Library of Congress Cataloging in Publication Data

Ward, Kathryn B.

Women in the world-system.

Bibliography: p.
Includes index.
1. Women—Developing countries—Social conditions.
2. Women—Developing countries—Economic conditions.
3. Fertility, Human—Developing countries. I. Title.
HQ1870.9.W36 1984   305.4'2'091724   84-8243
ISBN 0-03-069754-9 (alk. paper)

Published in 1984 by Praeger Publishers
CBS Educational and Professional Publishing
a Division of CBS, Inc.
521 Fifth Avenue, New York, NY 10175 USA
© by Praeger Publishers

456789 052 987654321

Printed in the United States of America
on acid-free paper

Foreword

It is most fitting that a book demonstrating the inter-relationship between the world economic system, women's status, and fertility behavior is published in the wake of the 1985 End Decade Conference on Women. In the appraisal of achievements accomplished for women over the past ten years in the area of conceptualization and research, Kathryn Ward's book is a landmark.

It is not that the past decade has neglected to draw attention to the economic and political forces that have shaped sexual inequality—a progressive step considering the overflow of past literature that grounded explanations for inequities in cultural forces. Recent years have also witnessed the raising of issues concerning the relationship of women to the new international economic order. However, the frame of analysis utilized in these studies, whether implicitly or explicitly comparative, focussed on the internal structure of nation-states. Research on the international effects of the capitalist mode of production on women's access to productive resources were very few in number and tended to be individually based case studies.

Kathryn Ward in this book presents us with the first cross-national systematic research on the specific effects of the world economic system—indexed by levels of foreign investment from and trade dependency on core nations—on women's economic status and fertility.

The conceptualization provided in this work, backed up by supportive empirical evidence, enables us to "make sense" of what heretofore have been contradictory findings regarding the relationship between nation-state economic development levels, women's status, and fertility. Seduced by the optimistic logic of modernization theory, it was difficult to understand why women's response to increasing levels of economic development was not consistently in the predicted "modern" direction. This is because national-level indicators of economic development, independent of international economic relationships, are not a sufficiently powerful predictor of women's condition. It is the qualitative contingencies that surround economic transformations at the internal nation-state level—in this case foreign investment from and trade dependency on core nations—that have also to be taken into account to fully understand what is happening to women in the process of development.

The themes that receive most attention in this book are the conditions of underdevelopment generated by the world economic system that place women relative to men in a disadvantaged situation in the competition for access to productive resources. As a result of the intensification of her marginalization from the productive process, woman pursues strategies of childbearing either because she is unable consciously to choose fertility reduction or because she may find such a reduction economically disadvantageous. Stripped of her economic/productive role, woman has to depend on motherhood performance for status and prestige and on her children's labor as a strategy for survival.

The concept of patriarchal relations is also emphasized throughout much of the book and serves to remind us of the presence of "actors" at work in perpetuating women's disadvantaged condition. At the same time it is equally clear that patriarchal manipulation directed at legitimizing and controlling what productive and reproductive roles are to be socially and economically acceptable for and to women are deeply rooted within the foundations of the mode of production. This is an important point to underline for those who naively attribute the disadvantaged position of women to practices of sex discrimination, and try to bring about improvement in her economic status without addressing structural factors that condition the production process.

The findings reported in this study point to clear linkages between the world economic system and women's share of economic resources. The effects of investment and dependency on fertility, however, show that previous relationships reported regarding the economic development/fertility equation are only slightly reduced when the influence of the world economic system and consequent income inequality are controlled.

Given such findings, what may we expect the policy implications to be?

It is difficult to conceive that policy action to rectify for women's disadvantaged economic situation in countries characterized by high foreign investments and strong dependency status could be forthcoming. Determination to act in this direction would involve interventions in exploitative international relationships that have a detrimental effect on women. It may be unrealistic to expect that many developing countries would act in that direction for the sake of women.

Some more hopeful possibilities regarding policies to reduce fertility that do not impinge on international economic relationships are suggested by the findings. I refer here to independent efforts that can be enacted to accelerate infant/child survival.

The findings indicate that the currently high levels of infant mortality could well undercut the desired effect that increasing levels of economic development and family planning programs could have in reducing the birth rate. High infant mortality levels, admittedly, are not an independent phenomenon, but are symbiotically related to conditions of underdevelopment, in general, and to the low status of women, in particular.

In the field of research and advocacy this book opens new horizons for the development and research community. The arguments pursued and results presented clearly call for the incorporation of indicators of investment and dependency status into the analytic framework of studies addressing the economic condition of women and her fertility behavior. As a corollary, there is a critical need to incorporate the "woman-dimension" into theory building on and analysis of world systems, differentiating between conditions of classical dependency and dependent development.

There is yet another sense in which this book marks a contribution—in this instance to modernization theory and to the field of women's studies. Recognition of the critical role of international economic relationships in shaping the internal structure of developing nations reaffirms the deep differences in the historical experience between the now-industrialized countries and those currently experiencing economic transformation under conditions of economic and political dependency. These differences outweigh by far the cultural diversities characterizing the two worlds. This book provides evidence of the impact that these historical differences have on the lives of women in developing nations—a fact to be remembered as one follows the paths of evolution of women in developing economies. It is precisely the recognition of such differences between the two worlds—known to exist but not as explicitly articulated as in this book—that has made a union between the women in development movement and the field of women's studies bereft with some difficulties.

Nadia H. Youssef
Senior Policy Specialist
Programme Development and
Planning Division, UNICEF

Acknowledgments

This book is dedicated to my late mentor, Jane Alison Weiss, of the University of Iowa. Through Jane's inspiration, work, and supportive tutoring, I grew to appreciate macro theories and the cross-national diversity of women's lives. Armed thus with an ecological and world-system perspective, I set out to explain the world of women. I can only hope that in Jane's absence I have done justice to her framework in explaining a small part of women's lives. Her spirit and memory have enabled me to pursue my research on both the good and bad days.

The research that formed the basis of this book could not have been completed without the support of persons at the University of Iowa and other universities who provided intellectual guidance after Jane's death and in my years at Southern Illinois University. Toby Parcel and Fred Pampel cochaired my dissertation committee. My other committee members—Charles Mueller, Jay Teachman, David Wagner, and Nancy Hauserman—provided additional advice.

I also acknowledge the network of Jane's friends at Stanford who were important sources of support for this research. Rachel Rosenfeld commented extensively and tastefully on most of the papers from and drafts of this manuscript. Other advice was given by Francisco Ramirez, Chris Chase-Dunn, Susan Olzak, François Nielsen, and Richard Rubinson.

More recently other colleagues have read and offered comments on several drafts of this book. Michael Timberlake and Sally Hacker read parts of the manuscript, while Linda Grant and Davita Silfen Glasberg graciously consented to read the entire manuscript.

I would like to thank Beverly Morber, Beth Forristall, Christina Huskey, Feri Sarikhani, and Eunice Prosser for typing various drafts. I would also like to acknowledge the support of Charles R. Snyder, chair of the department of sociology at Southern Illinois University, for the completion of this manuscript. I thank my editor, Lynda Sharp, for her strong interest in the topic of women and development within the world-system. Finally, the following women provided important support and encouragement for me while I was writing this book: Patricia S. Ward, Rose Arnhold, Kazuko Odani, Seanza Prasai, Shirley Nuss, and last but not least J. Lynn Turner, D.V.M.

Parts of this manuscript originally appeared in "The Economic Status of Women in the World-System: A Hidden Crisis in Development," in Crises in the World-System, edited by Albert Bergesen (Beverly Hills, Calif.: Sage Publications, pp. 117-39). Other parts of the manuscript appeared in "Toward a New Model of Fertility: The Effects of the World Economic System and the Status of Women on Fertility Behavior" (Working Paper 20 on Women in International Development, East Lansing: Michigan State University, Office of Women In Development).

Contents

Chapter

List of Tables

List of Figures

xv

This book is dedicated to

Jane Alison Weiss (1943-1981):

feminist, mentor, and friend.

1
Introduction

Recent inquiries into cross-national development and fertility often have focused on two seemingly separate areas: the effects of socioeconomic development on the status of women (i.e., women's access to social, economic, and political resources, relative to men's access); and anticipated changes in fertility during economic growth in developing countries. Studies with the first focus generally have shown that the status of women declines in the process of economic development (Boserup 1970; United Nations 1980). A "trickle-down" effect from men to women does not occur during development. Rather, women's traditional sources of livelihood are disrupted without a sex-equitable redistribution of the new economic and social resources generated by economic growth (Papanek 1976; Tinker 1976). Statistical studies with the second focus show that, despite economic growth, many developing countries have undergone only a small fertility decline over the last ten years and that a few countries actually have had an increase in fertility.

I will argue that these two areas of inquiry are inextricably bound and can be most readily understood within the context of the world economic system. It is within this system that women compete for access to valued resources relative to men and make decisions about their fertility. Recent research has demonstrated that the developing and developed nations interact within an international division of labor.[1] This international system disproportionately enhances the wealth of developed nations at the expense of the developing nations (Wallerstein 1974). This capitalist system emerged during the sixteenth century and has grown to encompass all regions of the world

1

within an international division of labor. Some of the early capitalist nations to emerge in this system became the core nations, while other regions and nations became incorporated as peripheral areas. Still other countries became the semi-periphery, or intermediaries between the core and periphery.

The interaction of the various geographical areas in this capitalist division of labor led to the phenomenon of under-development rather than development for the peripheral areas. Underdevelopment was the result of trade dependency and foreign investment, which created disruption of indigenous economies, reduced relative rates of economic growth, and heightened income inequality (Bornschier, Chase-Dunn, and Rubinson 1978; Bornschier and Chase-Dunn in press).

The structural disruption of the local economies meant that raw mineral extraction, cash cropping, and other forms of production were often oriented toward the core nations. In return, peripheral areas received processed goods from the developed areas. Over time, with growing populations, the peripheral regions were unable to provide enough jobs and goods relative to their populations. Further, capital generated by mineral extraction and cash cropping flowed to elites in the periphery and elites and populations in the core. Thus, this capital was underutilized in development efforts. Finally, such patterns of dependency and investment resulted in higher levels of inequality as the resources generated by economic growth were unequally distributed among the population of the periphery and between the core and periphery.

A more recent phenomenon within the world-system is the increasingly central role of core or transnational corporations (TNCs) in generating what some researchers have called depend-ent development (Cardoso and Faletto 1979; Evans 1979). This form of development relies heavily on foreign investments in factories engaged in local production of previously imported goods and/or production for export. Although this type of development is seen by some as a panacea for the problems of peripheral areas within the world-system, other researchers have argued that the long-term consequence of this type of investment is also underdevelopment (Bornschier and Chase-Dunn in press). Production in the import substitution factories, for example, often is oriented toward the consumption needs of elites and not toward the population as a whole. TNC plants oriented toward production for export have an additional dis-advantage. Products of these plants, particularly electronics components and microchips, are not manufactured for use in the periphery, but instead are returned to the core, where they are added to core consumer products (North American Congress on Latin America [NACLA] 1977; Siegel 1978/79).

In studying these socioeconomic phenomena, however, most researchers in the development and world-system perspectives have ignored two important social consequences of these processes: the declining status of women and the high levels of fertility. The major hypothesis I advance in this book is that the intrusion of the world-system through foreign investment from and trade dependency on core nations has operated to reduce women's status relative to men's. Underdevelopment and the export to developing countries of Western definitions of women's proper place have produced a double burden for women in developing nations. Men and the TNCs often define women's proper roles as reproducers and unpaid subsistence laborers within the domestic sphere. As a consequence, women experience not only the material consequences of underdevelopment and the disruption of their traditional sources of economic livelihood, but also limited access to the new mode of monetary or wage labor production introduced by the world-system.

This process is illustrated in a number of developing countries. When agricultural technology has been introduced, most typically only men have had access to new techniques, crops, and credit, even though women have been the primary agricultural producers (Boserup 1970; Tinker 1976; United Nations 1980). Women traders have been relegated to local trade routes, while men control national and international trade relations (Mintz 1971). Finally, with the introduction of capital-intensive investment and new industries from the core countries and corporations, women who previously produced similar goods in labor-intensive cottage industries have lost their markets. They are not subsequently incorporated into the industrial labor force. Although some women are now being utilized in the TNCs' global assembly line via the export-oriented plants, the unstable nature of these plants in the competitive world economy does not promise long-term job security for these women (Grossman 1978/79; Ehrenreich and Fuentes 1981; Fernández-Kelly 1983).

If women are denied access to the limited number of new jobs introduced by investment and dependency, how are women acquiring their economic subsistence, especially those women responsible for their own support or a substantial proportion of the household income? Many women now are found in the lower echelons of the service sector in domestic service or, alternatively, in the informal or unpaid sector (International Center for Research on Woman [ICRW] 1980a, 1980b). In these

sectors women provide much of the household income by subsistence agriculture, hawking foods and goods, and petty
trading—work that is an extension of their household labors.
Yet this existence is tenuous if women lack access to the monetary
economy. With the growing number of female-headed households
around the world (30 percent on the average), most women are
in a precarious economic position (Buvinic, Youssef, and Von
Elm 1978). Therefore, as a result of the conditions introduced
by dependency and investment, women's economic status relative
to men's has declined. This is particularly true in the areas
of the world marked by high levels of trade dependency and
foreign investment—primarily the peripheral areas.

A second major hypothesis I advance is that women's reduced
status during underdevelopment has impeded the anticipated
decline of fertility. The level of fertility in developing nations
remains high compared to fertility of the developed nations.
A fertility decline has not occurred in part because women in
developing nations, with reduced leverage over their home and
work environments as a result of underdevelopment, often can
gain socioeconomic status only through childbearing (Dixon
1975; Newland 1977). Further, under the conditions of underdevelopment, the value of children remains high (Hout 1980).
Women, through their own unpaid labor and their children's
labor, can generate up to half of the income of the household
(ICRW 1980a). Also, the world-system can prevent a decline
in fertility through the creation of conditions conducive to
high levels of infant mortality and income inequality—factors
that operate to maintain high levels of fertility. Consequently,
women may be less inclined to use family planning programs
because family limitation is neither a conscious choice nor a
socioeconomic advantage to them or their families (Coale 1973).
Thus, foreign aid and investment programs that include manda-
tory family planning projects can have contradictory effects
on fertility (Mass 1976). These projects are likely to be less
than effective, especially if the investment programs generate
conditions of underdevelopment, declining status of women,
and high value on children.

This book examines how the world-system affects the economic status of women and, in turn, how these two phenomena
affect fertility. This research represents the first empirical
examination of the specific effects of the world-system on the
economic status of women and fertility. Chapter 2 provides an
overview of the major theoretical perspectives of development
and the world-system. The specific relationships among trade
dependency, foreign investment, the status of women, and

fertility are then articulated. Chapter 3 describes the sources of cross-national and aggregate data, variables, and analytical techniques used in this research. Results of larger empirical analyses on the economic status of women and fertility are presented and discussed in chapters 4 and 5. Chapter 6 draws conclusions and considers the policy considerations of the study.

NOTES

1. Many definitions exist for "developed" and "developing" nations. I chose to distinguish between the two groups of countries on the basis of criteria cited by Todaro (1981). He argues that developing nations in contrast to developed nations are characterized by low levels of living (income, health, and education) and productivity. These characteristics are accompanied by high rates of unemployment and underemployment, population growth, dependence, and vulnerability in international relations.

Theoretical Overview

This chapter provides an overview of recent trends in
research on development, the world-system, the status of women,
and fertility. First, I review theories of development, dependency, and the world economic system. This section ends with
a discussion of why patriarchal relations or patterns of male
dominance over women should be incorporated into discussion
of the world-system. Second, I summarize literature on the
status of women in developed and developing countries and
outline linkages with the world-system. A particular emphasis
of this section is the economic status of women in the agriculture,
industry, and service sectors, including the newly emerging
role of transnational corporations (TNCs) in women's employment.
Women's access to educational, political, and organizational
resources is also examined. Third, I discuss the relationships
among the world-system, the status of women, other social
factors, and fertility. In general, my argument is that the
status of women, or women's access to economic resources relative
to men's, is negatively affected by the intrusion of the world-
system and patriarchal relations. In turn, women's fertility
remains high, especially if during development women are denied
access to alternative forms of socioeconomic status.

THEORIES OF ECONOMIC DEVELOPMENT

Three frameworks have characterized research on socioeconomic development in sociology: the social differentiation or
linear stages theory, the modernity theory, and the dependency

or world-system theory (Portes 1976). Social differentiation theory postulates a unilinear process of development, wherein newly developing nations merely need to follow the social and economic path of developed nations. Developing nations are supposed to move from traditional and ascriptive modes of social and economic organization toward achieved modes of modern social and bureaucratic organization. Proponents of this model have held that, through appropriate application of capital and technology from developed countries, developing countries would be able to generate industrial and economic development (Portes 1976; Todaro 1981).

Modernity researchers, on the other hand, have focused upon the "psychological complex of values" derived from developed nations that brings about modern thought and individual behaviors conducive to development. As Inkeles and Smith (1975, p. 3) have noted, "Nation building and institution building are only empty exercises unless the attitudes and capacities of the people keep pace with development." Researchers using this perspective argue that newly introduced modern institutions need people with modern values and behavior to run them effectively. The adoption of these modern values and behavior can take place through either exposure to modern economic and political institutions (for example, factories) or independent exposure to these values during the process of development.

More recently, these two approaches have been criticized for the omission of structural factors, for ignoring the consequences for economic growth of the adoption of certain modern values within a setting of underdevelopment, and for ignoring the effects of development on the status of women relative to men (Papanek 1978; Portes 1976; Tinker 1976). First, the linear stages and modernity theories, by defining development as an individual nation-state phenomenon, do not incorporate suprastructural relationships among various actors that take place within the context of the world-system. Second, the impact of international factors capable of mediating the effects of development on economic and sociocultural relations within nations has been ignored. Because of underdevelopment, the population remains for the most part unexposed to modern institutions (Frank 1966; Chase-Dunn 1975; Rubinson 1976). Third, the introduction of modern ideologies sometimes encourages practices that stymie development efforts. For example, consumption-oriented ideologies directed toward the purchase of foreign products do not generate widespread demand for local products or production facilities (Portes 1976). Finally, these perspectives have assumed that the status of women automatically will be improved during socioeconomic development. Women are assumed to gain increased access to economic resources and to benefit from adoption of modern values pertaining to the roles of women. As Boserup (1970), Nash (1980), and others note, women in developing countries have lost status during development. Patriarchal ideologies frequently have been reinforced rather than challenged.

Social differentiation and modernity theories are clearly inadequate because they do not include the emerging structural contingencies and consequences of the world economy for development efforts and the status of women. The failure of these theories to explain increasing underdevelopment and the declining status of women in developing countries suggests that we should look to the world-system perspective as a more inclusive framework.

WORLD-SYSTEM

The emergence of world-system theory as a major perspective in studying development took place in the 1960s, when theorists began to examine the failure of industrial development policies designed to increase industrial and economic growth in developing countries. Frank (1966) articulated one of the primary tenets of this perspective: Developing nations would never follow the developmental path of developed nations because of the exploitative nature of relationships between these two groups of nations. The economic growth of developing countries was dependent on their relationship with the developed nations or regions. For example, industrial production in peripheral regions of developing nations was oriented toward the metropoles or centers of developing and developed nations rather than being oriented around indigenous economic development.

This position was expanded by Galtung (1971), who proposed that economic development in developing nations was mediated through the trade dependency relations between developed and developing nations. In the course of imperialism and the eventual spread of the world-system, center (or core) nation-states established bridgeheads (harmony of interests) for trade with the center elites of peripheral nations. As a consequence, center nation-states, in collusion with the elites of the periphery, were able to bring about a concentration of trade partners wherein peripheral nation-states traded predominantly—if not exclusively—with a single core nation-state. Further, commodity concentration occurred. Instead of pursuing commodity diversification, peripheral nation-states were encouraged to trade or produce for export only one or two commodities. Last, center nations encouraged elites in peripheral states to export raw materials, with the center nations providing finished goods. In peripheral nations, this form of trade restrained the development of indigenous production facilities and encouraged the growth of trade structures skewed toward the export of raw materials and the import of finished goods. Such trade relations created trade dependencies on center nation-states and the overall impoverishment of the periphery, resulting from the flow of capital and resources to the elites and workers in the center.

In related research, Wallerstein (1974, 1979) examined the origins and nature of the world-system. He proposed that in the sixteenth century a major economic revolution took place with the emergence of the global capitalist economy. Within the world-system, nation-states interacted within an international division of labor. The first capitalist states to emerge became core nations, fueling their economic development at the expense of peripheral colonies and nations. Core nations, needing raw resources and markets for their expanding industries and commodity production, were able to control and dictate the economic operations of the world-system. At the same time, socioeconomic institutions of peripheral nations and colonies underwent significant disruption as the new mode of economic and monetary production, marked especially by the introduction of raw material extraction and cash crops for core markets, entered local subsistence economies. In turn, processed goods from the developed nations were brought into the economies of developing nations. Over time, most regions of the world were brought into the world-system.

Thus, the rise of the world-system became synonymous with the spread of capitalist commodity production and an unequal division of labor throughout the world, thereby generating new economic resources for competition among nation-states, populations in indigenous economies, and other actors, such as transnational corporations (TNCs) (Chase-Dunn and Rubinson 1979). Not all these resources were distributed equally. Chase-Dunn (1975) argued that, under this division of labor, foreign aid and investments actually had negative consequences for long-run economic growth and exacerbated income inequality in the periphery. These consequences occurred because resources generated by investments flowed out of the country to the core nations and corporations and were not reinvested within peripheral nations.

In a more recent formulation, Bornschier and Chase-Dunn (in press) have outlined three types of intrusion or investment by core countries and corporations operating within the world capitalist economy. The first type, which they have labeled classical dependence, takes the form of raw mineral extraction and cash cropping that is prompted by core nations and representatives of transnational corporations (TNCs) in peripheral areas. In turn, the developed countries provide finished goods. The second type, import substitution, evolved through the discontent of developing countries with traditional development strategies. Import substitution in manufacturing was promoted, e.g., where local elites in peripheral nations sought foreign investment in manufacturing plants to produce products for the local markets but primarily for the elites. Here TNCs invested in new plants or bought out already existing plants in semiperipheral or peripheral nations (Müller 1979). This form of investment has remained the largest share of TNC investment of manufacturing.

The third and a more recent type of investment trend has been the emergence of the global assembly line of TNC plants oriented toward production for export (NACLA 1977). Here TNCs have invested in labor-intensive manufacturing plants that produce electronics, textiles, shoes, and so forth. Production begins in capital-intensive plants within developed nations. Piecework is shipped to labor-intensive plants in developing nations. Then goods are returned to developed nations for finishing touches. The TNCs pay tariffs only on value added abroad. Thus, the manufacturers are able to take advantage of the cheap labor costs (particularly female labor) and free trade zones in developing countries (Froebel, Heinrichs, and Krege 1980). This last trend has marked the beginning of a new or global division of labor with a detailed division of production among nations and areas (Braverman 1974; NACLA 1977). Further, innovation and control over technology have remained in the hands of TNCs (Bornschier and Chase-Dunn in press).

The latter two types of investment by core corporation have represented the emergence of the process of dependent development (Cardoso and Faletto 1979; Evans 1979) wherein some economic growth takes place with the introduction of core corporations within developing nations. However, Bornschier and Chase-Dunn (in press) argue that, like the classical form of economic dependence, the new form of dependent development also has generated underdevelopment. Under these conditions, developing nations have failed to utilize fully their capacity for economic growth and redistribution of wealth.

In their empirical examination of the cross-national relationships between core corporation intrusion, economic growth, and income inequality, Bornschier and Chase-Dunn found that TNC investment in manufacturing was indeed related in the long run to lower levels of economic growth and to higher levels of income inequality for developing countries. Thus, in the short run, investment and aid that flow into a developing country can have positive effects on economic growth. Over time, however, a high concentration of foreign investment stocks creates structural distortion or blockage of the economy, heightened income inequality, and lowered economic growth, particularly for the more developed nations in the periphery (Delacroix and Ragin 1981; Bornschier, Chase-Dunn, and Rubinson 1978; Bornschier and Chase-Dunn in press). For example, specific sectoral investment in agriculture, extraction, or manufacturing has had a negative effect on economic growth because capital-intensive production often is oriented toward the elites in developing countries and both the elites and populations of developed countries (Bornschier, Chase-Dunn, and Rubinson 1978; Bornschier 1978; Bornschier and Ballmer-Cao 1979).

Intervening Mechanisms

A major criticism of the world-system approach has been the neglect of the intervening mechanisms by which underdevelopment is generated or mediated from foreign aid/investment and trade dependency (Portes 1976; Skocpol 1976). Recent research, in particular from the Zurich Multinational Corporation Project, has begun to fill this gap (Bornschier and Ballmer-Cao 1979). By specifying the role of TNCs in the manipulation of the world and indigenous economies, researchers have found that specific forms of investment and internal nation-state mechanisms mediate the effect of the world-system on economic growth and income inequality.

Three mechanisms that affect the distribution of power within a society intervene in the relationships among foreign aid/investment, economic development, and the structure of income inequality within developing countries: the state, the structure of the labor force, and urbanization. A strong core state can bring about development and decrease income inequality by controlling the economy, by dictating terms of foreign investment, and by redistributing resources, while simultaneously protecting and furthering the interests of economic organizations based within the state. Further, the state can equalize the access of the population to educational institutions (Rubinson 1976; Bornschier and Ballmer-Cao 1979; Meyer et al. 1979). Weak government or state structures in peripheral nations can result from relationships with core nations (Rubinson 1976). In the past, peripheral states often were unable either to control the extent and nature of core intrusion (e.g., by dictating the terms for transnational corporation investment) or to protect indigenous economies from the fluctuations of world markets. Recent research has suggested that some weak peripheral and semiperipheral states have reversed these subordinate relationships and have become stronger vis-à-vis core states. This dialectical process is related to the degree of the nation-state's incorporation within the world-system, rather than to its level of economic dependence (Ramirez and Thomas 1981). This research, however, focuses on the effects of economic dependency on state strength.

As a result of investment and dependency, economies in developing countries have failed to generate enough jobs to keep pace with population growth (Todaro 1981). Symptomatic of this phenomenon has been the extraordinary growth of employment in the service or tertiary sector at the expense of the manufacturing or secondary sector (Evans and Timberlake 1980; Kentor 1981; Timberlake and Kentor 1983; for alternative specification see Fiala 1983). In developed countries the growth of the manufacturing sector preceded the growth of the service sector. The developing countries, however, have shown a pattern of excessive growth in the service instead of the manufacturing sector. Foreign investment and trade dependency have encouraged adoption of capital-intensive industries that create relatively fewer industrial jobs for an ever-increasing supply of workers. Similarly, such forms of investment in agriculture have released a major part of the agricultural labor force. As a consequence, a large supply of workers had migrated to the urban areas in search of work, but many are relegated to the service and/or the informal sector (Portes and Walton 1981). Thus, TNCs' capital-intensive investment does not generate a long-term industrial employment but leads to the growth of the service sector. Hence surplus workers from the agricultural sector must seek employment in the limited industrial sector, the overcrowded and less productive service sector, or the informal sector. The latter sector buttresses the low wages paid by TNCs. Employers assume that workers will meet their subsistence requirements both through meager wages and by using services provided in informal sectors, for example, street hawkers or unpaid labor within the home (Deere 1976; Tinker

1976). As jobs in the paid labor force are scarce, economic
growth is reduced because resources for future development
are not generated and income inequality is increased for the
majority of the population.

Other intervening labor-force mechanisms, including the
bargaining power of labor, bureaucratization, and the power
sharing of elites with technical and industrial experts, mediate
the effects of underdevelopment. Strong labor organizations,
for example, influence the share of the economic surplus going
to the population rather than to the elites or corporations. In
a like manner, the growth of bureaucracy and elites' sharing
of power with experts spreads the economic surplus and limits
the growth of hierarchical authority, including the power and
decision-making ability of TNCs (Bornschier and Ballmer-Cao
1979).

The final internal mechanism is the overurbanization of
developing nations (Kentor 1981). Investment dependency
decreases the role of the industrial labor force, thereby leading
to the disproportionate growth of the service and informal
(nonmonetary/subsistence) sectors. Given the "city-lights"
phenomenon of rural-to-urban migration, overurbanization
occurs without commensurate urban economic development and
sufficient employment opportunities (Todaro 1981). Hence,
the growth of urban areas in developing nations does not
generate the same positive economic effects that urbanization
produces in the already developed nations (Timberlake and
Kentor 1983; Timberlake in press).

In summary, world-system researchers have found that
foreign investment and trade dependency from and dependency
on developed nations have had deleterious effects on economic
development, internal structures, and income inequality in
developing nations. Two additional phenomena of the world-
system remain to be explored: the role of patriarchy and the
status of women.

Patriarchal Relations of the World-System

In general, the previous theoretical work and descriptions
of the world-system and the pursuant international division of
labor have been focused on male economic and social institutions.
Another major component—patriarchal relations—must be added
to these explanations. I define patriarchal relations as the
institutionalized patterns and ideologies of male dominance and
control over resources that have generally empowered men to

define the productive and reproductive roles and behavior of women (Hartmann 1976; Saffioti 1978; Sokoloff 1980). These relations are divided into two parts, material and ideological: (1) the actual mechanisms by which men dominate and control existing resources and the sexual division of labor relative to women, and (2) the ideologies that justify the resulting sexual inequality. The strength of patriarchal relations in each mode of production is a major determinant of the sexual division of labor and the relative status of women or women's access to or relative control over valuable resources.

Patriarchal Mechanisms

Since the rise of the world-system, most women have lived within the confines of a feudal or precapitalist mode of production in the home vis-à-vis the larger capitalist society (Boulding 1977; Saffioti 1975, 1977, 1978). Men as a group have been incorporated into the new mode of economic or commodity production; male elites have controlled the means of production. Until recently the majority of women have remained within the precapitalist mode, the household form of production and reproduction (Hartmann 1976). With the expansion of economic production from the home to the marketplace within developed nation-states during the twentieth century, women in developed countries have gradually been drawn into commodity production. They also have continued their unpaid labor within the home (Waite 1982). With the incorporation of developing countries into the world-system, most women in these countries have remained within household production (Boserup 1970) and have lacked access to the new economic resources generated by the intrusion of the world-system.

Within each mode of production, patriarchal relations have served to define what productive and reproductive roles are socially and economically acceptable for women (Rubin 1975; Rosaldo 1980; Eisenstein 1979; Chodorow 1979). In more recent times, women's acceptable roles have ranged from equal and active participation in productive processes outside the home, accompanied by low levels of reproduction in socialist nations, to relegation to household production and high levels of reproduction in certain Arab countries (Leghorn and Parker 1981). Eisenstein analyzes the interrelationship between patriarchal relations and the prevailing mode of production for a variety of sociocultural settings as follows: ". . . patriarchal relations take place as patriarchy precedes capitalism through the existence of the sexual ordering of society which derives from the ideological and political interpretations of biological difference. In other words, men have chosen to interpret and politically use the fact that women are the reproducers of humanity" (1979, p. 25).

Each mode of production generates a division of labor that also shapes the sexual division of labor within a society (Deere, Humphries, and Leon de Leal 1982). Depending on what resources are available in each mode of production, the definition and allocation of roles between women and men may differ. For example, Deere and Leon de Leal (1981) note that with the intrusion of the world capitalist system of production in agriculture, greater flexibility in traditional patterns of the sexual division of labor in Colombia and Peru emerged. Women in the least affected areas remained within traditional forms of household production, while women whose husbands have joined the wage labor force became involved in agricultural production. This more flexible division of labor, however, did not mean the emancipation of women. Instead, as Deere and Leon de Leal note, women's agricultural participation was viewed as part of their subsistence labor within the home, indicating that ". . . the development of capitalism takes advantage of and reproduces the continuing subordination of women" (1981, p. 360).

Women's involvement in the mode of production and the sexual division of labor can determine the reproductive strategies of women and the households within which they reside (Deere, Humphries, and Leon de Leal 1982). If women are relegated to subsistence production in the home and the reproduction of the labor force through childbearing (and rearing) in rigidly patriarchal societies, women pursue strategies of childbearing (Safilios-Rothschild 1982). Hence, the international division of labor under the world capitalist system affects the operation of patriarchal relations through the mode of production within societies and through the sexual division of labor. Women's productive and reproductive roles continue to be defined by men and delimited by the prevailing mode of production.

In contemporary times, the operation of patriarchal relations is crucial to the maintenance of capitalism within nation-states and within the world-system (Saffioti 1978). Production and consumption needs within capitalist societies and within the larger world-system are manipulated by the capitalist elites to avoid crises of capitalism. This manipulation is implemented via patriarchal control over when work, motherhood, or both roles are economically necessary and socially legitimate. The dialectical relationship between women's productive roles outside the home and reproductive roles within the home facilitates this process because the socioeconomic value of women's production in the paid labor force reinforces the value of women's production and reproduction within the home (Sokoloff 1980). If women have no or limited access to economic resources outside the home, their power within the home to control their fertility vis-à-vis men's power to do so is weakened. These dialectical relations thus become an important mechanism of capitalist equilibrium when women are needed as workers outside the home or as childbearers or as both workers and mothers. In this manner, the relative crises of supply and demand for workers can be resolved.

These definitional manipulations of women's dual roles have been used within all nation-states. For example, during World War II, U.S. and European women, at first encouraged to enter the male-dominated sectors of the labor force under the guise of patriotism, then were systematically returned to the home during the 1950s. Only through the growth of economy and the pursuant demand for female labor were women in developed countries drawn back into the female-dominated sectors of the labor force (Oppenheimer 1970; Milkman 1976). Now they are incorporated as an essential component of the capitalist world-system of commodity production. Much of the postwar economic expansion of developed nations thus can be attributed to the expansion of the service sector and women's increased work roles.[1]

With the incorporation of women into the global assembly line, many women's work and reproductive roles are directly shaped by the international division of labor and patriarchal relations. Within developing nations, TNCs have seized upon the use of cheap female labor to remain competitive in such industries as electronics. First, the global assembly line represents a newly emerging, detailed division of labor that is incorporating women as a major source of labor. Second, within each plant a patriarchal atmosphere of male authority is reproduced to maximize the production of the women workers and to insure the perpetuation of the local patriarchal order in the society (Grossman 1978/79; Elson and Pearson 1981a, 1981b; Ehrenreich and Fuentes 1981; Lim 1983b).

Although some researchers have argued that such employment benefits women by liberating them from patriarchal constraints and by modifying fertility norms (Lim 1983a, 1983b), Elson and Pearson (1981b) argue that a dialectic between capital and gender emerges in such plants. The global assembly line may intensify, decompose, or recompose gender subordination (1981b, p. 157). The effects of these plants may decompose the subordination of women by undermining traditional family structures and by delaying marriage/childbearing. Yet such subordination is intensified through the patriarchal atmosphere generated in the plants and is recomposed through the authority of men in the managerial positions in these plants. For example, women are encouraged to make themselves commodities for the marriage market through participation in beauty pageants sponsored by the companies. However, if women marry or become pregnant while working in the plants, they are fired or pressured to quit (Grossman 1978/79; Elson and Pearson 1981a). Once again, patriarchal relations interact with the mode of production to perpetuate control and definition over women's productive and reproductive lives.

Over the last century patriarchal relations have had international and national forms and consequences. On the international level, as peripheral nation-states became more integrated within the world-system and thereby become exposed to prevailing world cultural trends, patriarchal relations in developing countries were also reinforced by the exportation of Western definitions of women's proper place within the domestic realm from the core to the periphery (Van Allen 1976; Saffioti 1978; Elu de Lenero 1980). Emerging during the Victorian era, this ethnocentric version of women's domestic roles as "breeders and feeders" led planners from core nations to ignore women's often significant socioeconomic and political roles within peripheral nations. This ignorance resulted in negative material consequences for women because this ideology (along with local patriarchal ideology) reinforced women's exclusion from the new socioeconomic institutions (Boserup 1970; Boulding 1977). More recently, because planners lacked knowledge of women's roles, development and economic programs frequently have been targeted for men only (Tinker 1976). As a result, men have had nearly exclusive access to the new economic resources generated by the world-system.

Within nations, the export of these Western definitions of women's roles has frequently reinforced indigenous patriarchal elements and the impoverishment of women (Leghorn and Parker 1981). In addition to the favored economic and political status accorded to males, TNCs and developing countries—in order to forestall labor unrest—have stressed Western and local patterns of passivity for women workers in the global assembly line (Grossman 1978/79). Further, women, who increasingly are becoming the sole support of households in developing countries, have been denied access to the monetary economy, thereby creating greater poverty (Buvinic, Youssef, and Von Elm 1978). Thus, as Saffioti (1978) notes, the theme of women's primary place within the domestic realm has been used to blame women both for their seemingly lower economic contributions and for espousing values inimical to development.

In core nations, as women have gained greater access to economic resources, the influence of patriarchal relations is less apparent. At the same time, patriarchal relations have persisted as a dominant force in women's lives. Women continue to experience the burdens and contradictions of the double day, in which they work outside the home and still are responsible for children and most of the unpaid labor performed within the home (Eisenstein 1982; Waite 1982). In peripheral nations, women have lost control over the new social and economic resources generated by the intrusion of the world system. Nevertheless they continue to have responsibility for childbearing and for much of subsistence and household production.

Thus, patriarchal relations, in conjunction with the world-system and the internal structures of nation-states, have important implications for the economic status of women and for fertility. The economic status of women, defined relative to the contingencies of capitalism and patriarchal relations, depends on the relative economic need or demand for women's work or motherhood roles. As the demand for female labor outside the home fluctuates, fertility behavior is affected.

STATUS OF WOMEN

In recent years the relative status of women in economic development has received closer scrutiny (Boserup 1970; Youssef 1974; Friedl 1975; Dixon 1975, 1978b; Blumberg 1978; Rogers 1978; Whyte 1978; Rosaldo 1974, 1980). The concept usually has been defined primarily in economic terms. I define the status of women as women's access (relative to men's) to economic resources. Secondary components of women's status consist of women's access to educational, political, and organizational resources. The following discussion is divided into three parts: (1) the theoretical rationale for this definition and for examining the status of women in the world-system, (2) a survey of women's status during development, and (3) the linkages between the world-system and women's status.

Theoretical Perspective on Women's Status

Theoretical formulations of the status of women in development have emerged from studies of women's status in public
and domestic spheres (Rosaldo 1974; Sanday 1974). These
authors have argued that in the process of economic transformation from the precapitalist to the capitalist mode of production,
men came to control resources in the public domain. Women
remained in the domestic arena attending to private production
or household and childrearing duties. Status in the public
domain, then, came to be defined in terms of control over
economic, social, and political resources that existed completely
out of the home.
One of the best delineations of women's status in relation
to the public sphere is Sanday's (1974, 1981) formulation of
women's cross-cultural status differentials. Sanday concluded
that women's status was the highest in the public domain (male
sphere) when, in particular, women had control over material
products outside of the domestic sphere and development
generated a demand for female products. Additional dimensions
of status included women's political participation and women's
organizations that operated to protect women's economic or
social interests, such as trading territories (Sanday 1974,
p. 192). The important relationship between these dimensions
noted by Sanday (1974) and Blumberg (1976, 1978, 1979),
among others, was that women's control over material products
was a necessary but not sufficient source of female status and
power in the public domain.
These dimensions are crucial for defining women's status,
but the economic status of women also is dependent on the
nature of resources within the public domain. Women may
appear—as they do in many developing countries—to have high
status in the public domain because of high labor-force participation and control over subsistence agriculture and regional
trade. Sanday (1974, 1981) has noted that women have lost
status within the public domain if men are able to achieve an
external sphere of control over valued resources (perhaps as
a function of war). I argue, however, that the intrusion of
the world capitalist system has led to a change in the nature
and types of resources in the public domain. Commodity production introduced by the world-system has become the major
external sphere of control for men relative to women. Men as
a group have greater control over the socioeconomic resources
introduced by foreign investment and trade dependency. Thus,
where women and men once were engaged together in production

within the home, the advent of the new commodity form of production has facilitated greater male access to and control over the monetarized and industrial sectors of the economy in a new sexual division of labor (Hartmann 1976; Young 1981). Likewise, the differentiation of educational and political institutions under capitalist development has enabled men to gain control over these valued resources. Meanwhile, during underdevelopment, women have remained essentially within precapitalist forms of production and have had variable access to the resources generated by the new mode of production only according to the needs of the capitalist system, for example, within the global assembly line. Further, women generally have been precluded from positions of political power. Thus, these relations of patriarchal control over women have been reconsolidated with the advent of core-periphery relationships among nation-states (Saffioti 1978) or the intrusion of the world-system in the periphery.

If we redefine the public domain as consisting of the educational, economic, political, and organizational resources generated by the various facets of the capitalist mode of production within the world-system, we have a basis from which to compare the status of women with that of men. This comparison also allows certain patterns to be detected when, under the influence of the world-system and patriarchal relations, women remain within precapitalist modes of production, for example, in extensive involvement in agricultural production, or women have limited access to educational, labor-force, and political resources relative to men. The important distinction between women and men, then, is what type of capitalist or employment resources members of each sex can gain access to for leverage over their environment. If access is limited, women can use only children or subsistence production resources for achieving status (Newland 1977; Youssef and Hartley 1979).

Status of Women: A Survey

Since the International Women's Year in 1975, an increasing number of studies have indicated that in general women continue to lag behind men in every facet of status, although there are differences by regions, forms of economic organization, and state structures (United Nations 1980). In the past researchers have assumed that economic growth and development led automatically to higher status for women (Inkeles and Smith 1975; Mauldin and Berelson 1978), but the newer studies have con-

cluded that women in developing countries have usually suffered
severely negative consequences during underdevelopment
(Boserup 1970; Papanek 1976; Tinker 1976; Youssef 1976;
Boulding 1977; Saffioti 1978; International Center for Research
on Women [ICRW] 1980a, 1980b; United Nations 1980).[2] These
studies show that underdevelopment usually has operated to
lower women's status in developing countries as measured by
women's access to economic, educational, political, and organizational resources. The next sections discuss these various
dimensions of women's status. First, women's employment is
examined in developed countries, and then there is a more
detailed discussion of women's work in developing countries
in the agricultural and trading sectors and in industrial, service,
and informal employment. Second, women's access to educational
resources is examined. Third, the institutional and legislative
problems of women's political status are outlined. Last, women's
organizational resources such as feminist movements, organizations, and unions are discussed.

Trends in Employment

    During the 1950-1970 period, the proportion of women
employed outside the home in the world increased from 31.2
to 35.0 percent (United Nations 1980). This trend, however,
is expected to continue only for Latin American and developed
nations. Women's current levels of participation are likely to
decline in Asia and Africa. The major reason for this decline
is the failure of developing economies to generate jobs at a rate
faster than population growth (Todaro 1981). In addition,
because of underdevelopment within the world-system, these
figures conceal significant gender employment and sectoral
disparities (see Table 2.1).

Employment in Developed Countries

    A substantial number of women in developed countries
have entered the labor force since 1950. By 1970, 45 percent
of nonfarm European women were working, compared with 43
percent of women in the United States. These percentages
are even higher in state-controlled economies where the state
has attempted to incorporate the female labor force (International
Labor Office 1977; Lapidus 1978; Szabady 1977). The growth
exhibited over the period 1950-1970 was related to industrial
expansion by developed countries and demand for female labor
in the growing tertiary or service sector. In addition, the
decline in the number of single women workers (because of a

TABLE 2.1

Women in the Labor Force: Participation Rates and Relative Share, 1950-1970

Region	Participation Rates (%)		Female Share of Labor Force (%)		% of Female Labor Force in Service		% of Female Share in Service	
	1950	1970	1950	1970	1950	1970	1950	1970
Europe	29.4	30.5	33.0	36.0	35.0	48.0	39.0	44.1
Eastern Europe	41.3	45.0	42.0	45.0	20.0	32.0	39.4	51.4
Northern America	24.0	30.3	28.3	37.0	71.0	77.8	40.0	46.1
Latin America	12.7	13.5	18.0	21.4	53.0	67.2	34.0	38.4
Africa	28.0	25.2	33.0	33.0	12.1	18.0	33.2	34.0
Northern Africa	4.4	4.7	7.0	8.6	8.0	13.0	13.1	14.3
Asia	26.0	30.0	29.0	34.4	37.0	38.0	14.0	25.0

Source: Compiled by author from employment data from International Labor Office (1977).

higher marriage rate) was more than compensated for by an increase in the number of married women workers with children (Oppenheimer 1970; Blake 1974; Stolte-Heiskanen 1977).

Since a sex-specific demand for female labor was created by the growth of the service sector in the developed economies, the growth in women's employment opportunities has meant unequal employment of women and men. The expropriation of unpaid home production under the expansion of capitalism merely transplanted "women's work" to paid labor in the service sector (Sokoloff 1980). Consequently, women workers were channeled into clerical, service, and sales occupations and were excluded from administrative and managerial positions in the evolving gender division of labor under monopoly capitalism (Oppenheimer 1970; Blake 1974; Weiss, Ramirez, and Tracy 1976; Stolte-Heiskanen 1977; Coser 1981; Young 1981). Furthermore, significant pay disparities have persisted between women and men (Blake 1974; United Nations 1980).

Finally, there are additional indirect consequences of the world-system and patriarchal relations for women's work in developed countries. In an unstable global economy, women's work in developed countries may be constrained by the demand for cheap female labor in developing countries. Given recent downturns in the economies of developed countries, there is increasing competition by TNCs for international markets. Women who are in the marginal and production-oriented sectors of the economy have lost their jobs to the overseas movement of manufacturing plants seeking cheap female labor in developing countries (NACLA 1977; Grossman 1978/79; Ehrenreich and Fuentes 1981; Nash 1983; Robert 1983). Thus, the relative economic status of women in developed nations can have an important influence on the status of women in developing countries through the export of female segregated industries needing cheap labor and the material consequences of prevailing ideologies from developed countries on women's proper place (Safa 1981).

Employment in Developing Countries

Because of the undernumeration of women's economic contributions in developing countries by official statistics, it is difficult to convey an accurate picture of women's economic role (Fong 1975; ICRW 1980a, 1980b). Since 1950 there have been regional variations in women's share of the labor force and participation rates. In 1975 Africa had the highest participation rate at 45.8 percent, followed by Asia, Latin America, and the Middle East with 11.4 percent (ICRW 1980b). These officially reported participation rates also vary between rural and urban areas (Boserup 1970; Youssef 1974). Women's participation in both areas is uniformly low in the Middle East and Muslim countries, where women are secluded in agricultural and home industries (Papanek 1971; Dixon 1978b). In Southeast Asia, women's participation is high in both sectors. Women are utilized in labor-intensive agriculture, services, and cottage and factory industries (Mazumdar 1979; Jahan 1979b). Latin American women have low rates of rural participation in capital-intensive agriculture but higher rates of urban participation in domestic service, factories, and clerical work. Finally, African and Indian women show high participation rates in rural sectors through subsistence agriculture and own-account trading. Women's participation in nonagricultural employment in the urban areas is relatively low.

These economic patterns, as well as women's informal-sector roles, suggest that women in developing countries contribute a substantial share to their economies and to development efforts (Boulding 1977; ICRW 1980a, 1980b). These official figures, however, do not fully represent women's total economic contributions and status. First, high participation rates are not always equivalent to high status. In comparison to men, women may have diminished access to the new resources generated by investment and trade. Second, to calculate women's total economic contribution, one must include their role in the informal or subsistence sector.

During underdevelopment, foreign investment and trade dependency have led to a disjuncture between public and private production. Patriarchal relations have redefined women's economic roles as the less important sphere of production within the new gender division of labor based on the positive social evaluation of women's reproductive roles. As a consequence, women's work roles must be examined vis-à-vis the classical and new types of foreign investment and dependency.

Agricultural Employment

During periods of classical economic dependence (high commodity concentration and less diverse trade structures) and when women were subsistence agricultural providers, men received greater preference for cash or commodity crops introduced by colonial officials and TNCs (Boserup 1970; United Nations 1980; Seidman 1981). While women have remained in the fields using the same implements, men have obtained greater access to new agricultural techniques and technology. Where developed nations and TNCs have encouraged new technology for export food processing, men have controlled this technology and women have lost their jobs (Boserup 1970; Jahan 1979b; Chaney and Schmink 1980; ICRW 1980a, 1980b). For example, with the introduction of rice rollers from Japan, many women were displaced from rice hulling production (Tinker 1976). Finally, men were recruited almost exclusively for raw mineral extraction by colonialists and TNCs (Boserup 1970; Mueller 1977).

Trading Employment

The opening of new trade relations within the world-system has negatively affected women's regional trading routes in both rural and urban areas in the Caribbean, Africa, and Southeast Asia. This effect occurred because men acquired control over the more remunerative international and national trade routes (Boserup 1970; Mintz 1971; Simms and Dumor 1976/77; Van Allen 1976; Jain, Singh, and Chand 1979; Joseph 1980; Papanek 1979a, 1979b). As Ward (in press) has noted, many women traders have participated in the trading enclave economy. This was a cheap transportation and distribution network between the larger world economy and the subsistence sector within a country (Simms and Dumor 1976/77; Sudarkasa 1977). Unfortunately, increased contact with the world economy has increased economic uncertainty for women traders, because their existence has become interdependent with the world economy, the economic diversity of the country's trading patterns, and local patriarchal relations. Women traders have become increasingly dependent on others for large amounts of capital to finance their trade operations. For many women, the increased need for capital has meant greater dependency on men and, in particular, their husbands. Other women have resisted such dependency by forming women's economic associations for savings and credit (Simms and Dumor 1976/77; Robertson 1976; Jules-Rosette 1982). With women's relegation to subsistence agriculture and regional trading, however, women's trading and agricultural activities clearly have not been enhanced by contact with the classical forms of economic dependence within the world-system.

Industrial Employment

Most of the new foreign investment in developing countries has been in manufacturing. As noted by Bornschier and Chase-Dunn (in press), two types of foreign investment in manufacturing by core countries have emerged in the new economic dependence: import substitution and processing for export (off-shore sourcing). These two types of investment have different short-run effects on women's access to industrial employment. In the long run, however, I predict that both forms of investment will lower women's access to employment. Over both time spans, investment for import substitution has lowered the proportion of women in manufacturing because of import of capital-intensive technology from core nations for factories and a preference among employers for male workers (Chinchilla 1977; Miranda 1977; Shapiro 1980). This capital-intensive TNC and local investment has created a lower number of jobs relative to the supply of displaced agricultural workers or those seeking urban employment in developing countries. These workers must enter the service and/or the informal sector (Evans and Timberlake 1980; Kentor 1981; Lunday and Timberlake in press; Fiala 1983). Given the paucity of paid jobs and the strength of patriarchal relations, men have preference for the few available jobs. Further, women's cottage or labor-intensive industries frequently have been unable to compete with products of the new factories. Women also have been denied employment in new industries, thereby seriously disrupting women's employment opportunities in Central and Latin America and in India (Chinchilla 1977; Arizpe 1977; Mazumdar 1979). When women workers have been displaced from previous activities or migrated to the urban areas, they thus have not moved into factory work, but into the tertiary or service sector (Chaney and Schmink 1980).

TNC Employment

The other type of foreign investment under new economic dependence, export processing, still constitutes a smaller proportion of manufacturing investment compared to import substitution. Nevertheless, this type of investment has a disparate impact on the employment of women relative to men. In Latin America and in Asia, women have experienced greater access to the global assembly line in labor-intensive industries, such as clothing or electronics. Meanwhile, previously observed trends toward declining employment of women in industry in the short run have been reduced. Up to 90 percent of the employees of these industries are either female or minorities (Ehrenreich and Fuentes 1981; Fernández-Kelly 1983). These women workers, I argue, now constitute important mechanisms for stabilizing competitive crises in the global assembly line.

Why were women targeted as employees in these plants, and what have been the consequences of this targeting for long-term women's employment and national development? The TNCs targeted female workers because of the lower female wage rates. TNCs found that women workers would accept earnings up to 50 percent lower than men's (Elson and Pearson 1981b). Further, TNCs and host governments argued that female workers were much more likely than men to be passive and nonorganizing workers. Concessions by host governments on the enforcement of protective labor legislation also provided an incentive for investment (Grossman 1978/79; Ehrenreich and Fuentes 1981; Safa 1981; Fernández-Kelly 1983). Finally, local patriarchal relations of control over women were replicated within the factories by structuring the plants as one big family with father figures and male managers wielding authority over women workers' habits and lives (Elson and Pearson 1981a, 1981b; Grossman 1978/79; Lim 1983b). Because of the demand for these female workers, TNCs have employed more than 2 million women (Ehrenreich and Fuentes 1981).

Over time, however, this type of employment has been less than beneficial for women in terms of stability, wages, unions, and host countries. TNC production for export has been notoriously unstable in the competitive world economy. Consequently, thousands of women workers have been laid off during international recessions. Further, turnover in these plants has been high because of harmful working conditions and firings related to marriage or pregnancy. One can easily imagine the effects on eyesight, for example, of peering through a microscope for eight to ten hours a day for two to three years. After such experiences, many women no longer have the good eyesight needed for employment (Grossman 1978/79). Finally, if women workers threaten to unionize or strike for higher wages, the TNCs move their runaway plants to other, more receptive countries, for example, from South Korea to Malaysia or Indonesia. As a consequence of the employment instability in TNC plants, Ehrenreich and Fuentes (1981) estimate that more than 9 million women now have worked in the global assembly line.

Researchers and TNC officials have argued that women's wages benefit the status of women and the development efforts of the country (Lim 1983a, 1983b). Closer examination, however, reveals that many women's wage levels barely have met subsistence levels—even for their own countries. For example, Grossman (1978/79) notes that in Indonesia, the starting monthly wages for women are approximately $19; after two years of employment the salary rises to $29 per month. The basic monthly expenses for one person (including sleeping space shared with four or more people, food, and transportation) are $26. Therefore, although company officials have boasted of the consumer purchases made by their employees, i.e., mopeds, closer examination of the data shows that most of the women employees have been living on marginal wages. Further, many of these women are expected to send part of their already meager earnings back to their families (Salaff 1981; Fernández-Kelly 1983).

Efforts to organize women workers to improve the level of wages and working conditions have been met either with force or with threats to move the TNC plants. At the same time, the governments in developing countries have provided less than adequate protection for female workers. For example, in a number of TNC plants, efforts to unionize women workers have been met by thugs who put down strikes and union organization (Grossman 1978/79; Ehrenreich and Fuentes 1981; Safa 1981). Likewise, sometimes protective legislation for women workers suddenly has disappeared if a TNC has indicated an interest in locating in a developing country. Thus, women's organizations seeking better wages and working conditions have been stymied by antiunion attitudes of TNCs and sudden removal of protective legislation by their host governments (Elson and Pearson 1981a; Rosenberg 1982).

Finally, development planners and TNC officials have boasted of the positive indirect effects from TNC investment for a host country: training of the labor force, capital for development, and reduction of the unemployment rate. As Siegel (1978/79) and others have noted, these promised benefits rarely have materialized. Training in TNC plants frequently has not been transferable to other industries. As a result, thousands of women workers have held TNC employment and then have been laid off without transferable job skills—a situation that is a direct consequence of the detailed international division of labor. Further, profits generated by such investment generally have flowed out of the country instead of being used for development (Müller 1979; Bornschier and Chase-Dunn in press). Thus, the only major source of money generated for development from these plants has been the women's meager wages. The overall employment situation in developing countries has been affected only minimally by this labor-intensive investment, because the TNCs have generated a demand for women workers previously uninvolved in the labor force rather than unemployed workers. Thus, as was predicted by earlier research on the relationship between TNC investment and economic development, only short-run benefits have accrued to host countries and women workers. In the long run, economic development has been hampered (Bornschier and Chase-Dunn in press; Timberlake and Kentor 1983; Lim 1978; Siegel 1978/79).

Meanwhile, numerous women have been subjected to hazardous working conditions, have received low wages, have learned consumer-oriented values (relating to cosmetics, clothes, mopeds, and so forth). These large doses of Western ideology about passive females have reinforced local patriarchal relations and ideologies. Finally, where do these displaced women workers go? Some go into prostitution (Neumann 1978/79); still others go into the service or informal sectors.

Service Employment

In developing countries, the primary means by which women participate in the service sector is domestic service. Other common occupations are food production, trading, small-scale production, sewing, clerical work, and retail sales. The service sector is quite heterogenous and includes women who hawk single cigarettes and sticks of gum in the streets or serve hamburgers in fast food establishments (Tinker 1976). Women's work within this sector frequently blends into the informal sector of employment (ICRW 1980b), where jobs are characterized by no or minimal wages and little or no social protection (Portes and Walton 1981; Portes in press).

Women's involvement in the service sector has its origins in women's domestic production within the home. During development and underdevelopment, many of women's domestic labors are brought into the marketplace to exchange for wages. Further, many of women's domestic activities are conveniently combined with work brought into the home for pay, such as laundering or sewing. The only difference between the two activities is that women are only paid for the work brought into the home (Jelin 1977, 1980).

These domestic linkages, however, present problems in raising women's economic status relative to men's. In general, young women in developing countries are domestic servants until they marry, gaining little training or education for mobility into other occupations. Further, domestic service, either as a servant or in home activities, is poorly paid (Jelin 1977). Wages often consist only of room and board for many young women migrants. As a consequence, patriarchal relations of subordination are reinforced by women's patterns of service-sector activities, because women, compared to men, still do not have equal access to the new service-sector jobs generated by development.

Among the service workers in the modern economy, women are less likely to be clerical workers in Africa but more likely to be in these occupations in Latin America. Women traders in

Africa frequently are denied positions in the retail and whole-
sale sales sector of commerce (Boserup 1970). Researchers
have noted that women's limited educational opportunities are
an impediment to women's service-sector participation. Since
there is a relative oversupply of educated male workers, men
are frequently given preference for jobs (Tinker and Bramsen
1976; Matyepse 1977; Standing 1978; Chaney and Schmink 1980;
ICRW 1980b). In fact, Asian men have taken over women's jobs
in the service sector (Papanek 1979b).

Informal Employment

Given these trends of women's displacement from the agricultural, trading, industrial, and sometimes service sectors,
where are women in developing countries seeking their economic
livelihood? Women's displacement from other sectors has resulted
in the economically disruptive growth of both the service and
informal sectors, the latter defined here as subsistence agriculture, domestic/cottage industries, food preparation, small-scale
trading, and unremunerated labor performed within the home
(United Nations Economic Commission for Africa 1975; Awoskika
1976; Jahan 1979b; Schmink 1977; Shapiro 1980). According
to estimates, the informal sector is quite large in the urban
areas of developing countries, encompassing 53 to 69 percent
of urban workers (ICRW 1980b). Further, until recently women
rarely have been considered in research on the informal sector
even though women constitute the majority of workers in this
sector. They make up an estimated 46 to 70 percent of the
informal sector in Latin America and only a slightly lower percentage in Southeast Asia (Tinker and Bramsen 1976; ICRW
1980b, p. 68; Cho and Koo 1983; Koo and Smith 1983). This
disparate treatment is interesting in light of the acknowledged
importance of this sector for the operation of the world-system
(see Portes in press).

Women's informal-sector participation is tied to the processes
of underdevelopment generated by foreign investment and trade
dependency. Saffioti (1978) has argued that under core-
periphery relations, the growth of precapitalist activities such
as service or domestic types of work occurs. This work is
primarily women's work that contributes to the reproduction
of the core-periphery relations through the reproduction of
the labor force, use production within the home, and infrequent
work for wages according to the mode of production. Women's
informal-sector activities also allow the elites or capitalist class
to pay lower wages to those who work outside the home—the
hidden assumption being that workers will make up the difference

through the use of subsistence production of their wives and children (Deere 1976; Jelin 1977, 1980; Meillassoux 1981). In fact, Schmink (1977) argues that the extraordinary increase in the service sector noted by Evans and Timberlake (1980) was generated by the participation of women in the service and informal sectors under dependent development.

At the same time, these trends in the informal labor market mean that women have experienced decreased access to modern jobs generated by the world-system. Women's mobility in leaving the informal sector is limited relative to men's (Arizpe 1977; Chaney and Schmink 1980; ICRW 1980b; Jules-Rosette 1982). In fact, even within this sector, men have control over the better jobs (Wachtel 1976; Papanek 1979b). Finally, women, in particular women migrants and heads of households, in this sector are much more likely to live in poverty than are other workers. Wages, if any, are less than 45 percent of men's (Buvinic, Youssef, and Von Elm 1978; ICRW 1980a). Consequently, disruption of female informal-sector activities, in combination with declining economic opportunities in the monetary sector, places women in developing countries in a critical economic bind.

The economic pressures on women are particularly notable for two reasons. First, because of the increasing poverty of developing countries, many families have disintegrated compared with earlier times where families remained intact. As was mentioned before, a growing number of households in these countries now depend on female heads—on the average, over 30 percent of the households (Papanek 1979b; Joseph 1980; Buvinic, Youssef, and Von Elm 1978). The preference for male workers has limited increasingly women's economic options. Second, often the only resources available to women to provide leverage over their environment are their children (Newland 1977). This limited leverage hinders the lowering of fertility rates, since women view children as economic assets. In addition, informal-sector participation is highly compatible with childbearing, but it is less remunerative in terms of familial support than modern-sector employment (Blumberg 1978; ICRW 1980a). Even so, by working with their children, women can contribute over 50 percent of household income (Papanek 1979b; ICRW 1980a), thereby providing a hidden prop for the economic system of developing countries (Boulding 1977).

Overall, women's economic status has declined, because of the incorporation of the developing nations within the world-system. Women have little or no access to resources and have been relegated increasingly to the informal sector during underdevelopment. Women's access to other resources, such as education, likewise has been limited.

Education

For women in developed nations, economic growth has led to an overall increase in educational opportunities (Blake 1974; Weiss, Ramirez, and Tracy 1976; Stolte-Heiskanen 1977; Ramirez 1981). In general, women have gained increased access to education at the primary, secondary, and tertiary levels relative to men's. Economic development, however, has not produced equal educational access for women in developing nations. Many of the newly literate are men. Women remain less literate than men in Asia, Africa, and the Middle East (McGrath 1976; Tinker 1976). Although in Latin America women had reached parity with men at the primary and secondary levels by 1970, women in Asia and Africa lag behind even at the primary level. At the secondary and tertiary levels, women's share of education is even lower: 26 percent and 28 percent of tertiary enrollments for Africa and Asia (McGrath 1976). Because of increasing population pressures and underdevelopment, these nations have been unable to meet the demand for educational facilities (Todaro 1981). As McGrath notes, this problem particularly affects women because "equal education for women is hampered by a whole set of mutually dependent ideas and traditions that define and limit the female role. In developing countries, the acute shortage of educational facilities, in combination with a belief that boys should be educated first, effectively excludes many girls" (1976, p. 37).

The growth of educational opportunities in developed countries has had an important influence on the growth of female labor-force participation and the legitimizing of women's work (Weiss, Ramirez, and Tracy 1976). Education provides credentials for access to occupations. In fact, the growth in demand for female labor actually has been a growth in demand for educated female labor (Oppenheimer 1970). At the same time, aggregate growth in female education has not led to the coordination of women's degrees with actual job opportunities (McGrath 1976). Women are still encouraged to take "female" subjects in schools rather than pursuing studies in the sciences or other male-dominated fields (Dixon 1975; Coser 1981; Sanzone 1981). Thus, females' increased levels of education have perpetuated patterns of sex-typed jobs (Oppenheimer 1970; McGrath 1976).

In contrast, the gender education differentials in developing countries mask qualitative differences and the influence of patriarchal assumptions: Women's education is more frequently oriented toward domestic roles than toward skills for surviving in the monetarized economies or for increasing agricultural productivity (Boserup 1970; McGrath 1976; Tinker 1976; Van Allen 1976; Boulding 1977). Also, women's education may not provide access to jobs other than in the rural, agricultural, or informal sectors of the economy (Papanek 1976).

Political Status

The political status of women can be evaluated in two ways: (1) women's access to and integration within political institutions, and (2) legislation. Women frequently gain access to political institutions through suffrage. Even though most women have the right to vote in developing countries (except for seven Moslem countries), Chaney (1975) indicates that the political situation of women is constrained by women's traditional roles and underdevelopment. In a later work, Chaney (1979) found that economic development has not meant automatic changes in the political status of women. For example, Latin American countries with the highest gross national products were among the last to grant women the right to vote. Further, nearly universal suffrage has not produced the anticipated integration of women into government. After surveying the world political situation for women, Newland notes: "The near universal recognition of women's political rights and the strength of their voting numbers in many countries are nowhere reflected in their direct role in government" (1979, p. 100).

Worldwide, women have been integrated into political institutions only in times of crisis or through familial affiliations (Van Allen 1976; Chaney 1979; Epstein 1981a). Although a handful of women have gained access to the highest levels of government as prime ministers in Israel, Great Britain, Portugal, Norway, and India, the integration of women into all levels of political institutions has been limited. For example, most women cabinet ministers have dealt with "soft" issues, such as health, welfare, or education (Newland 1979). Consequently, those cabinet posts of a few women at the higher levels of government have had only a minimal influence on the government and women's issues (Sanzone 1981). Women's relative participation in legislative bodies has grown at a snail's pace since 1950 (Epstein 1981a, 1981b; Sanzone 1981).[3] As a result, women are not proportionately represented within most governments. Instead, women appear at the lower levels of bureaucratic and administrative positions (Newland 1979; Epstein 1981a).

It is not surprising, given these avenues of integration, that women frequently have viewed political participation as an extension of their traditional female roles of caretaking and mothering. On the one hand, this perception has led to the phenomenon of the supermadre (as it is termed in Latin America)— defined as the view expressed by many women that the country is essentially one big family (Chaney 1979).[4] Further, this perception, inspired by patriarchal tradition, does not necessarily mean that women are more politically conservative than men. Instead, it can mean that even women with records of political activity view politics as an unworthy pursuit compared with issues of economic survival (Chaney 1979; Jacquette 1980).

In developed countries, equal rights legislation and laws pertaining to women's right to control their bodies have proliferated over time (United Nations 1980; Sanzone 1981). In a review of family legislation in developed countries, Kamerman and Kahn (1978) found that most of the fourteen countries surveyed had implemented some type of policy to alleviate familial constraints on working women through provisions for maternity benefits, work leaves, and child care. In contrast, other countries (such as France, Hungary, and the German Democratic Republic) have provided higher levels of family allowances to encourage women to have children (Lapidus 1978; Westoff 1978; Kamerman 1979). Still other countries, such as the United States, have vague family policies (Kamerman 1979).

As women's participation in politics in developing countries is constrained by the demands of their economic roles and patriarchal relations, legislation to raise the status of women is similarly constrained and attenuated by prevailing conditions of underdevelopment. First, although women are beginning to acquire some semblance of rights in marriage and property law (United Nations 1980), so-called modern laws introduced through the world-system may disrupt women's traditional legal and economic power without giving them alternative forms of power (Nader and Collier 1978). For example, land reform frequently assigns ownership rights to men rather than women. Second, because most women work in unregulated sectors where equal employment laws are rarely applicable (Mazumdar 1979; Rosenberg 1982; United Nations 1980), their employment or economic subsistence rights are often ignored.

Perhaps the most discriminatory form of legislation is the selective enforcement of protective legislation. As Jahan remarks, "Whenever women demanded equal participation, the policy response was to provide them with special protective measures" (1979b, p. 63). The role of patriarchal relations becomes clear when one examines the consequences of protective legislation. Employers use protective legislation to deny women access to lucrative positions. In Peru, for example, after a 1957 protective labor law was passed, some factories refused to employ new women industrial workers (Chaney and Schmink 1980). The problem is compounded when women are denied additional training for new factory technology. Ironically, protective legislation that may exist is rarely enforced by a government when it encounters pressures from TNCs. Used together, the selective application of protective legislation and the denial of training block women's access to modern-sector work (Mazumdar 1979).

The legislation of most developing countries relating to women is a curious mixture of indigenous patriarchal attitudes and more recent provisions designed and enacted to make the country appear "enlightened" to the developed countries (Matyepse 1977; Safa 1977; Chaney 1979; Jahan 1979b; Newland 1979; Jacquette 1980; Lindsay 1980; Shapiro 1980). Researchers argue that legislation in this manner is used to the advantage of TNCs and local economic structures (Saffioti 1978). Meanwhile, if women's control over economic resources is disrupted, so-called progressive laws may hinder, rather than help, women's competition for jobs.

In general, growth in women's educational and employment opportunities has had little impact on increasing women's representation at the higher, more powerful levels of government. Epstein (1981a) suggests that women are still denied access to those elite tracks that lead to the highest governmental positions. The proliferation of legislation seeking to raise women's status has proven relatively ineffective in enhancing women's economic opportunities.

Women's Organizations

One means by which the female population can compete more effectively for educational, economic, and political resources is through organization. Parallel to the women's or suffragist movement in Europe and the United States during the nineteenth and twentieth centuries, a number of organizations specifically advocating changes in women's status have appeared in the developing nations (Blake 1974; Flexner 1975; Hurwitz 1977; McBride 1977). The movements to unionize women workers are examples of such organizations.

The impact of organization on the status of women in developed countries has been mixed. Although the women's movement in the United States and other developed nations has led to the adoption of legal reforms, these gains have not always come solely because of feminist pressures (Blake 1974; Freeman 1975; Sanzone 1981; Eisenstein 1982).[5] Still, national and local women's organizations have contributed to a diversity of changes on the national level through legislative reforms and on the local level through the implementation of grassroots projects regarding women's health care, education, and services to women (Freeman 1975). Overall, the women's movements in developed countries have contributed to a legitimization of women's rights to equal economic and political opportunities and to their control over reproduction.

Women's movements in developing countries have been for the most part middle-class reform movements (Van Allen 1976; Saffioti 1978; Chaney 1979; Jahan 1979b; Mazumdar 1979; Joseph 1980). Therefore, they have not touched on the daily lives of a majority of the women who may participate in nationalist movements and local economic organizations. Most legislative reforms generated by these movements are class-based: Equal educational and employment opportunities tend to affect only middle-class women; peasant and lower-class women are relatively unaffected.

As a consequence, many women seeking more than reform have participated instead in popular struggles against government and colonial dictators. In this sense, women have worked against basic structural inequalities. This form of participation has resulted not only in an integration of women within existing revolutionary movements, but also in an accelerated recognition (compared with the experience of women in the developed countries) of women's issues in Latin America (Flynn 1980), Africa (Van Allen 1976), Southeast Asia, and the Middle East (El Saadawi 1980).

Unlike the women's movements, women's economic organizations have long played a major role in the past success of women traders and farmers in the Caribbean, Africa, and Asia (Boserup 1970; Mintz 1971; Little 1973; Leis 1974; Lewis 1976; Van Allen 1976; Okonjo 1979; Joseph 1980). With colonial intrusion, however, many associations became unable to compete effectively with male organizations or TNCs for the new resources that were generated. Primarily, such groups were unable to gain sufficient credit or capital for members. Consequently, in some western African groups, traditional emphasis has shifted from exerting organizational control over a sector of the economy to acquiring appropriate "housewife" skills learned in "women's groups" (Van Allen 1976).

Unionization

The track record of unions in regard to the economic advancement of women has been dismal in most developed countries. Although efforts have been made to incorporate the female industrial labor force into unions in the United States, the female proportion of the nonagricultural unionized labor force has declined (Wertheimer 1977; Bureau of Labor Statistics 1980). The low proportion of unionized women has been related to the types of jobs women have entered. Clerical and service occupations are notoriously difficult to unionize. In contrast, Hartmann (1976) has traced how male workers in both developed and developing nation-states actively have sought to exclude women workers from traditionally male occupations and from unions. She concludes that the restrictive activities of capitalists and male workers have effectively blocked women workers from lucrative positions. Likewise, unionization among women in developing countries has been strongly discouraged by these nations' governments, sometimes with the help of international unions (NACLA 1977; Ehrenreich and Fuentes 1981; Siegel 1978/79). Governments in developing countries actively discourage unions, fearing TNCs might relocate their plants elsewhere. We must therefore conclude that unionization in conjunction with patriarchal relations of control generally continues to exert a negative influence on the ability of women to effectively compete for resources.

THE ECONOMIC STATUS OF WOMEN
AND THE WORLD-SYSTEM

Some Linkages

Women rarely have been included in research on the world-system (at either the international or the internal level). Therefore, an understanding of the linkages between the world-system and the economic status of women must be derived from previous theory. In general, higher levels of foreign investment and trade dependency found in developing countries relative to developed countries might be expected to lower women's access to economic resources, defined here as women's share of the labor force, economic sectors (agricultural, industrial, and service), and participation rate.

In past cross-national research, indicators of national economic development—such as gross national product per capita (GNP/c) and kilowatt hours per capita (KWH/c)—have shown a

positive or curvilinear association with women's share of tertiary
education and the labor force (Weiss, Ramirez, and Tracy 1976;
Ramirez 1981; Semyonov 1980; Nuss and Majka 1983). These
relationships might diminish, however, when indicators of foreign
investment and trade dependency are controlled. During underdevelopment, economic growth occurs at a lower relative rate,
and higher levels of inequality are created. In turn, the demand
for female labor at a given level of GNP/c fails to materialize as
expected. Thus, the effects of development on women's status
may vary over levels of investment and dependency. Furthermore, investment and dependency may more adequately reflect
the structure of the economy and the demand generated for
female workers than does GNP/c.

The effects of trade dependency and foreign investment
on women's economic status may vary according to the different
types of investment/dependency noted above: classical dependency and dependent development. With the operation of classical
economic dependency, the extent of commodity concentration
and the nature of the foreign trade structure are related to
women's employment. Where there is considerable diversification
of commodity and trade structures, significant growth in the
economic opportunities for women (their share of the labor force
or specific sectors) in developing countries occurs. If commodities are concentrated in either agriculture or raw materials,
women in developing countries lose economic opportunities other
than those in the subsistence agricultural or informal sector in
the long run. If, as expected, trade structures of developing
countries are oriented toward the export of raw materials and
import of processed goods, women will continue to have limited
access to jobs generated by this trade structure.

Some related types of investments, e.g., TNC investment
in agriculture and extraction, also are predicted to lower women's
share of the total labor force and the agricultural sector. The
investments in these sectors are marked by their capital-
intensive nature and demand for male labor. Hence, such investment should lower women's economic status.

During dependent development, investment in manufacturing
has come to constitute the largest share of overall TNC investments. One type of manufacturing investment is capital-intensive
and provides a limited number of jobs per investment dollar.
Given the scarcity of jobs for the population and the overall
preference for male labor (relative to the demand for female
labor), countries with high levels of TNC investment are predicted to have lower levels of women in manufacturing or
industry and in the overall labor force because of the intense

competition for jobs with other displaced (male) workers. Additionally, given the displacement of women workers from their traditional industries without the creation of new jobs in related industries, this displacement should contribute to women's smaller share of industrial employment. Further, considering the above relationships, we would expect the overall level of foreign investment to have negative effects on women's access to employment. These patterns are expected to follow the consequences outlined for the relative stocks and flows of foreign investment. Initially the flows might increase women's employment; but, over time, women's employment will decline because of the structural distortion of the economy introduced by trade dependency and foreign investment.

The other type of investment in manufacturing—production for export—constitutes a lesser share of TNC investment in manufacturing, but a greater number of female relative to male workers are used in these labor-intensive plants. As a consequence of the unstable nature of employment in these plants, we would expect to see short-run increases in women's employment and long-run declines in their employment as TNC plants move around the globe. Further, if TNC production in the core female-intensive industries is being shipped to peripheral nations, we should also find a long-run negative influence in developed countries on women's share of industrial employment and heightened female employment in the service sector. As underdevelopment continues, both women's and men's employment should be negatively affected by the investments in import substitution and production for export—phenomena already noted by Evans and Timberlake (1980) in their discussion of the extraordinary growth of the service sector.

Intervening Mechanisms

The influence of investment and trade dependency on the status of women in developed and developing nations also should operate indirectly through the intervening mechanisms discussed earlier: labor force characteristics, state strength, urbanization, educational resources of women, organizational capacity, and income inequality. (See Figure 2.1 for depiction of these relationships.)

The size of the labor force relative to the adult population and the size of the tertiary sector relative to the total labor force will lead to an increased demand for female labor. If the growth in the labor force fails to match the growth of population, women's economic opportunities for wage employment are nega-

FIGURE 2.1

The Influence of the World Economic System and Intervening
Mechanisms on the Status of Women

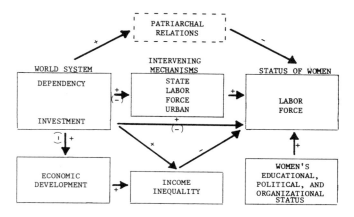

Note: This diagram should be viewed as a heuristic device,
not as a path model.

tively affected. One major avenue for women's entrance into
the labor force has been the service sector. Thus, recent
trends that have generated service-sector growth should enhance women's employment. Further, an increase in bureaucratization through the growth of clerical and managerial occupations
and elites' sharing power with experts should have a positive
influence on women's employment. Bureaucratization represents
a demand for female labor; the spread of power to experts
represents a more equal distribution of knowledge. On the
other hand, growth in labor's bargaining power should have a
negative influence on women's employment in developing and
developed countries, because of the active role of (male) labor
in excluding women from access to the labor force and, in
developing countries, because of high levels of unemployment.

Previous research has shown that a strong or mobilizing
state can affect women's employment opportunities through
incorporation of disadvantaged groups into the existing educational, economic, and political structures (Weiss, Ramirez, and
Tracy 1976; Sanzone 1981; Szabady 1977; Lapidus 1978; Ramirez
and Weiss 1979). Furthermore, state distribution of social
insurance program coverage varies among the developed and
developing countries. A strong state provides for maternity
pension benefits; weak states have limited or no coverage.

Women's leverage over their work and fertility roles may thus
be affected by state measures that determine the value of children
(Lapidus 1978; Westoff 1978; Mueller 1976). Finally, age at
marriage can be mandated by the state and local patriarchal
customs. Later age at marriage gives women a greater potential
for educational and labor-force experience in developing countries (Dixon 1975).

The level of urbanization has different implications for
women in developed and developing countries. While women in
developed countries have more access to the monetarized service
sector, women in developing countries frequently have been
relegated to informal-sector employment in urban areas.

The level of economic inequality within a nation is represented by income inequality. Though the relationship between
income inequality and the status of women is unclear, Semyonov
(1980) argues that heightened income inequality lowers women's
labor-force participation.[6] In contrast, it could be argued that
reduced female participation and economic opportunities during
underdevelopment lead to greater economic inequality, in that
resources are being unevenly distributed among the population.
Thus, in developing countries a higher rate of female participation in the monetary sector(s) should result in reduced income
inequality. To replicate Semyonov's results, however, I will
examine the effects of income inequality on the status of women.

Other facets of women's status may advance women's access
to economic resources. The state in developed countries has
incorporated women into expanded educational institutions, but
in developing countries significant disparities remain in the
population's access to educational institutions (as a result of
population pressures) and in women's meager share of educational
enrollments. Hence, if women's share of higher education is low
relative to men's, women are at a significant competitive disadvantage in the labor force. Further, the relative organizational
capabilities of women's organizations should differ between
developed and developing countries. Given the tradition of
female mobilization in developed countries, women's organizations
in these countries should be more effective in obtaining women's
access to resources than groups in developing countries. For
example, in the latter countries, many women's economic organizations have been unable to compete effectively with the new
contingencies of the world economic system. Finally, equal
rights legislation can help incorporate women within existing
economic institutions, thereby raising their economic status.

Finally, while patriarchy cannot be measured directly,
the influence of patriarchal relations on the relative status of

women can be inferred by examining the patterns of the relationships between the world-system indicators and the status-of-women indicators. If women's share of resources declines as a function of investment and dependency and the relative influence of intervening mechanisms within a nation-state, these findings are interpreted as suggesting the presence and influence of patriarchal relations, i.e., the domination of access to and control over resources by men as a group.

FERTILITY

The problems of high levels of fertility and population growth have attracted the attention of demographers and development researchers, who had expected levels of fertility to decline more rapidly with economic development in developing nations. This problem has forced researchers to reexamine the validity of the demographic transition framework and the role of economic development, international inequality, the status of women, and family planning efforts in the determination of fertility.

Demographic Transition

In the past, researchers have relied upon patterns shown in developed countries and their demographic transition to predict declines in fertility in developing countries (Coale 1973; Birdsall 1977; Knodel 1977; Mauldin and Berelson 1978; Tsui and Bogue 1978). In essence, initially high levels of births and deaths in developed countries were followed by a decline in the death rate during industrialization. A pursuant decline in the birth rate then resulted in reduced levels of population growth. From the pattern they perceived, researchers concluded that economic development was conducive to lowering fertility and to motivating populations to limit fertility.[7] Consequently, the path to lower fertility for developing countries was assumed to be through following the strategies of economic development used by developed countries.

Since there has been a moderate decline in fertility in Asia, but only a small decline in Latin America and no change in Africa (Tsui and Bogue 1978), the application of the demographic transition theory to developing nations is troublesome (see Table 2.2). As Teitelbaum (1975, p. 422) argues, numerous demographic and socioeconomic differences between developing

TABLE 2.2

Total Fertility Rates by Region, 1968 and 1975

Region	1968	1975
Africa	6,502	6,141
Asia	5,332	4,487
Latin America	5,526	4,909
Developed	2,361	2,128
World	4,635	4,068

Note: Rates are per 1,000 women over their lifetime.
Source: Tsui and Bogue 1978, p. 14.

and developed nations prevent the "natural or timely" decline of fertility. These differences occur because, for one thing, levels of demographic indicators differ widely from the experiences of developed nations. Mortality rates in developing nations declined more rapidly through the intervention of medical technology from developed nations, while fertility remained higher than earlier European levels. The rate of population growth has been higher over time for developing nations. This rate is bolstered by the hidden momentum of a disproportionately younger population. Another important difference is that crucial demographic and economic processes found in the developed nations have not occurred in developing nations, which lack the safety valve of international migration and have not generated increased occupational and educational resources for women.

Still other researchers have argued that the value of children in developing countries has remained high during development as a function of the perceived need for children through agricultural production and infant mortality. Likewise, Caldwell (1976, 1982) has noted that the crucial difference between fertility in developing and developed nations has been the influence of cash flows between child and parent. Social and economic transformations in developed nations resulted in cash flows going from parent to child and pursuant limitation of fertility. When the flow of cash is from child to parent, as is the case in developing nations, there is little incentive to limit fertility.[8]

In the absence of strong economic development effects, researchers have turned to a variety of internal "modernization" factors that have been found to affect fertility behavior. After reviewing the relative influence of numerous variables, Mauldin and Berelson (1978) used seven socioeconomic indicators to predict the change in the crude birth rate from 1968 to 1975. Beyond the influence of GNP/c, adult literacy—in the form of primary and secondary enrollments—was expected to depress fertility. Also, the life expectancy and infant mortality ratios were considered to be important, inasmuch as an increase in life expectancy leads to reduced fertility and a decline in infant mortality has a directly negative effect on fertility. An increase in the percentage of males aged fifteen to sixty-four years in the nonagricultural labor force was expected to lead to lowered fertility. Finally, an urbanization measure was used to represent the negative influence of urbanization on fertility. This array of social setting variables, plus family planning efforts, enabled Mauldin and Berelson to explain a substantial part of the crude birth rate decline.

In a similar effort, Tsui and Bogue (1978) incorporated measures of economic development, health, urbanization, proportion of females in agriculture, school enrollments, and family planning efforts in their prediction of changes in the total fertility rate (TFR) from 1968 to 1975. Once again, socioeconomic factors and family planning efforts had substantial independent effects on fertility.

These two studies are incomplete, however, in the omission or limited inclusion of variables concerned with the world-system and the status of women. Dixon (1978a), for one, argues that Mauldin and Berelson's estimates could have been improved if status-of-women variables had been included.

World-System

The characteristics of the world-system have rarely been considered in traditional analyses of fertility. On the one hand, most demographers, like earlier development researchers, have tended to view fertility and population growth as an individual nation-state problem (see, for example, Caldwell 1976). On the other hand, a few researchers have suggested that the economic interrelationships among nation-states are a major factor in the failure of economic development to generate the anticipated decline in fertility (Tilly 1978; Repetto 1979; Hout 1980). Arguing that "the high rates of population growth in

today's Third World countries will turn out to be less consequences of their own peculiar internal organizations than effects
of their economic relationships with the rich countries of the
West," Tilly (1978, p. 32) then goes on to suggest that relationships between trade dependency and fertility in developing
countries be examined.

Hout (1980) has examined the effects of classical economic
dependency on fertility in Latin America. He proposes that the
fertility decline has been impeded by the trade dependency of
developing countries on developed countries. He argues that
an intervening mechanism in this case is the socioeconomic value
of children, which remains high under the influence of dependency
relations. The overall relationship between development and
fertility is curvilinear, as development will not affect fertility
rates unless accompanied by a decrease in dependency relations.
Hout's specification of the model, however, does not include
measures of the value of children or the status of women. Thus,
he neglects intervening mechanisms by which the world-system
affects fertility.

The relationships between fertility and other forms of
investment under classical dependency, e.g., foreign or TNC
investment in agriculture or extraction, and under dependent
development, e.g., TNC investment in manufacturing or overall
levels of foreign investment, might be more indirect. If dependent development generates lower relative rates of economic growth
and heightened levels of income inequality, these conditions
might impede the anticipated decline in fertility. For example,
economic development would not provide the same negative
effects on fertility as are found in other nations. The large
number of people displaced by capital-intensive investment
frequently must find support and subsistence in the service
and informal sectors, where children are viewed as economic
assets. Further, the disparate distribution of resources under
income inequality results in only small incentives to limit fertility.
Researchers have found a stronger positive relationship between
income inequality and fertility than between fertility and the
level of economic development (Bhattacharyya 1975; Simon 1976,
1977; Repetto 1979). This strong relationship between income
inequality and fertility holds at both the international and
national levels (Repetto 1979). Thus, I argue that although
initial flows of investment might operate through economic
growth to reduce fertility, over time, the large stocks of foreign
investment leading to underdevelopment should limit the negative
effects of development on fertility. Additionally, the declining
status of women is another indirect avenue for the positive
effects of investment and dependency on fertility.

Status of Women

The relationship between the status of women and fertility has come increasingly under attention by researchers (Chaney 1973; Piepmeier and Adkins 1973; Dixon 1975, 1978b; Germain 1975; United Nations 1975b; Birdsall 1976; Westoff 1978). Most researchers have examined the relationship between women's labor-force participation and fertility (for summaries, see Kupinsky 1977a; Standing 1978).

A basic assumption of the following discussion is that the status of women (as previously defined) and that of children constitute two possible avenues for women to have leverage over their environment (Newland 1977). Therefore, a major determinant of fertility is the structure of opportunities for women, i.e., whether or not women have access to the new educational, economic, and political resources generated by development. Fertility is conditioned by the economic and social structure in which women reside (Davis and Blake 1956; Blumberg 1978; Safilios-Rothschild 1982).

Women in Developed Countries and Fertility

In developed countries there has been a gradual decline in fertility rates (Blake 1974; Stolte-Heiskanen 1977). Most researchers attribute this decline to later age at marriage, a lowering of marital fertility rates, expanding educational and occupational opportunities for women, and increasing availability of contraception (Teitelbaum 1975; Westoff 1978). Other research has examined the influence of more egalitarian gender roles and the incompatibility between motherhood and work roles (Rainwater 1965; Stycos and Weller 1967; Scanzoni and McMurry 1972; Dixon 1975; Hass 1972; Huber 1980). In the long run, as women in developed countries continue to receive higher levels of education and enter the labor force, fertility in developed countries should continue to decline and level out at replacement levels (Standing 1978; Huber 1980).

The only qualification to these specified relationships is the recent efforts by certain socialist and developed nation-states to encourage an increase in fertility through the provision of generous family allowances, maternity leaves, and housing incentives for women. These programs have been successful in raising the birth rate in Hungary and the German Democratic Republic (Lapidus 1978; Westoff 1978).

Women in Developing Countries and Fertility

The relationships between the status of women and fertility found in developing countries differ from those in developed countries. Relationships between education and labor-force participation and fertility, which are negative in developed countries, can be negligible or positive in developing countries (Kupinsky 1977a, 1977b; Standing 1978).[9]

Education. Within developing countries, education may have a negligible or positive influence on fertility. First, women have unequal educational opportunities and may not receive the knowledge or impetus to limit their families. Second, as noted earlier, education in developing countries does not lead to the types of occupations that depress fertility behavior (Dixon 1975). Thus, education might have a limited influence on fertility, although some research from Asia indicates that the level of education may be more important than labor-force participation (Hull 1977; Chaudhury 1979).

Labor Force. Researchers have concluded that women's relative economic contribution is an important intervening factor between economic development and fertility. Women's labor-force participation per se has only a negligible effect on fertility (Kasarda 1971; Kupinsky 1977b; Ware 1977; Standing 1978). As the level of economic development is an insufficient proxy for the economic status of women (Kasarda 1971; Dixon 1978b), the important distinction is the types of work that women engage in or have access to in the context of economies of developing countries.

A major reason for the negligible relationship between women's overall labor-force participation and fertility is that, in contrast to women in developed countries, the majority of women in developing countries have no choice between their motherhood (reproductive) and economic (productive) roles. Both are socially and economically necessary (Dixon 1975; Newland 1977). Such definitions of these roles are reinforced by the dialectical relationship between women's productive and reproductive roles. Where women have a lesser share of economic resources outside the home, they will be disadvantaged in regard to reproductive decision-making within the home. In such circumstances women receive much of their social status from their reproductive or childbearing roles, especially if their economic contributions are taken for granted but are perceived to be less important than men's work. Further, as Safilios-Rothschild (1982) has noted, in highly patriarchal societies women continue to have children until they have several boys to solidify their position and status.

Owing to these relationships, women's economic roles are, in large part, compatible with childbearing duties. Hence, we find that women engaged in rural agricultural cottage industries and other economic activities pursued from the home have higher fertility rates (Collver and Langlois 1962; Jaffe and Azumi 1960; Concepcion 1974; Ware 1977; Hass 1972; Dixon 1975, 1978b; Standing 1978). In contrast, women engaged in urban industrial production and in clerical and professional occupations have lower fertility. The difference between the groups is not only that between rural and urban living but also a variation in the extent to which women have access to the monetary sector.

Unfortunately, the sexual division of labor that is generated by the intrusion of the world-system rarely leads to a pursuant demand for female labor in the monetary sector. If women are relegated to the informal sector or remain in the agriculture or service sectors, as is the case in most developing countries experiencing underdevelopment, fertility will not be substantially lowered. These women will continue to carry out traditional and socially prescribed roles in which both work and motherhood are expected; they will not be exposed to new ideas, values, and information about family planning. Furthermore, children will continue to be valued resources, either because of child-parent cash flows or because of the fact that child labor is necessary to supplement family income (Caldwell 1976; ICRW 1980a). Due to these factors, women may not have the knowledge, status, or motivation to limit their fertility.

Consequently, if, as I believe, the influence of the world economic system through investment and dependency has been to decrease women's economic opportunities relative to men's and to maintain the value of children, then pressures arise that obstruct fertility reduction, phenomena not adequately represented simply by indicators of economic development. I propose that in countries with higher levels of investment and dependency, women will have lower economic opportunities in the modern or paid-employment sector. Furthermore, the value of children will remain high, because children provide part of the household subsistence income under these conditions. This is true especially with underdevelopment, which does not always generate increased opportunities for the wage earners (either female or male) of the household. Thus, some of the potentially liberating and antinatalist forces introduced by the intrusion of the world-system and different cultural norms can be counteracted by the consequences of underdevelopment and the declining or low economic status of women. The economic status of women should have an independent influence on fertility.

Political Resources. Although the political status of women is somewhat related to their economic status, the proliferation of legislation about women should have direct effects on women's fertility behavior (Chaney 1973; Dixon 1975; Germain 1975). First, if women are integrated into political and policy-making institutions, they not only serve as role models but also are in a position to implement measures that can enhance their own status. Second, legislative measures affecting the rights of women to equal educational and employment opportunities, maternity benefits, and child care opportunities can be strong antinatalist influences. If women are denied access to alternative resources because of restrictive practices, such as laws forbidding married women to work, they will utilize the other form of leverage available to them: children (Dixon 1975; Germain 1975; Newland 1977). Additionally, if nation-states legally raise the age at marriage, women's child-bearing years will be fewer. Conversely, state expenditures on family allowances that are substitutes for wages foregone may have a positive influence on fertility. Hence, the political status of women has an indirect, though important, influence on fertility behavior.

Organizational Resources. Women's organizations are a newly recognized resource for family planning and fertility limitation (Germain 1975; Bruce 1976; Dixon 1975, 1978b). These organizations can facilitate the dissemination of family planning information and generate social support for contraceptive practices. In addition, the economic organization and productivity of women workers can be enhanced through development projects based in women's organizations (Dixon 1978b). As a result, the role of women's organizations in the limiting of fertility can be substantial—directly by affecting contraceptive knowledge and usage and indirectly by facilitating economic and political opportunities for women.

Family Planning

When economic development did not bring about the anticipated decline in fertility of developing countries, development planners and demographers began to examine another option: technological solutions in the form of family planning programs. Unlike the proponents of the motivational approach of increasing economic development (Blake and Das Guptas 1978), the proponents of family planning argued that increased access to family planning programs might help alleviate the problem of population growth and bring about economic development (Todaro 1981; Tsui and Bogue 1978; Mauldin and Berelson 1978).10

Aggregate empirical analyses show that family planning program efforts have had an independent negative influence on fertility (Mauldin and Berelson 1978; Tsui and Bogue 1978). However, Dixon (1978b) has argued that these analyses are misspecified because of their significant omission of status of women variables that can explain a substantial and independent proportion of fertility behavior. This argument is important in light of the proposed linkages among underdevelopment, decline in the economic status of women, pursuant pressures toward fertility, and Coale's (1973) three determinants of fertility limitation.

Coale (1973) proposes that there are three preconditions for a fertility decline. First, the decision to limit fertility must be within the realm of conscious choice; that is, parents must find family limitation a socially acceptable practice. Second, family limitation must be seen as socially and economically advantageous. Finally, contraceptive knowledge and services must be available.

For women in developing countries, these conditions may be unmet. As Elu de Lenero writes:

It is difficult to achieve this [family planning and fertility decline], however, because humanity has spent all its history making women believe that their reason for existence is to have lots of children—and women believe it. Maybe the problem of population growth that now confronts the world can in part be attributed to having marginalized women from a more active social participation, and having confined them to a reproductive role (1980, p. 64).11

Under the sexual division of labor engendered by underdevelopment, women may find that family limitation is a less-than-viable strategy. Further, under these conditions, women, because of patriarchal definition of their roles and reduced access to alternative economic resources, may not have fertility limitation within the realm of their conscious choices (Sadik 1974; Tangri 1976; Dixon 1975; Germain 1975; Hass 1972; Safilios-Rothschild 1982). The pursuant power differentials within the family from the dialectic between women's productive and reproductive roles may lead to male disapproval of women's control over their fertility. Also, family limitation may not appear to be economically advantageous. High levels of infant mortality, increasing burdens on women's subsistence activities, and relegation of women to the informal subsistence sector may mean that children are still viewed as major economic assets (Ware 1977; ICRW 1980a). For these reasons, family planning services, even if available, may be underutilized or ignored.

A final linkage between the world-system, family planning, and fertility has also been noted. While the world-system through foreign aid/investment has contributed to the decline of the status of women and consequently impeded efforts to bring about fertility decline, these foreign aid/investment packages frequently have been granted only if they included funds for family planning efforts (Mass 1976). Thus, the effectiveness of family planning programs may be hindered by the deleterious effects that accompany foreign aid/investment.

I suggest that previous theoretical and empirical analyses of fertility are incomplete. Fertility behavior should be examined in the context of the world-system and the economic status of women relative to men. If these international and internal factors minimize the utility of family planning programs through underdevelopment, such technological solutions are likely to be ineffective.

If attention is paid to the possible interventions in the exploitative international relationships that impede development and in particular affect the status of women, family planning programs will be more likely to succeed. As Hout (1980) notes, economic development has only a minor influence on fertility unless accompanied by a change in dependency relations. Likewise, I argue that fertility will be little influenced by economic development and family planning programs unless the marginalization of women and perpetuation of the high value of children during underdevelopment are taken into consideration. The incorporation of women into development efforts, therefore, is a necessary component in the efforts to bring about a decline in fertility.

THE WORLD-SYSTEM, THE STATUS OF WOMEN, AND FERTILITY: SOME LINKAGES

Four sets of predictions can be set forth for analysis of fertility behavior: (1) the influence of the world-system and status of women on fertility; (2) the relative influence of social setting variables on fertility, controlling for the previous factors; (3) the relative influence of family planning program

FIGURE 2.2
The Influence of the World Economic System and the Status of Women on Fertility Behavior

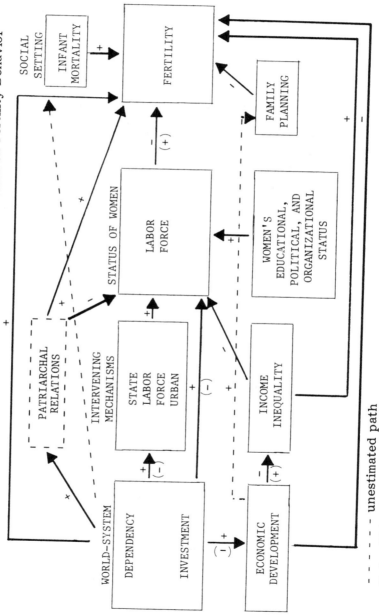

- - - - unestimated path

Note: This diagram should be viewed as a heuristic device, not as a path model.

53

efforts on fertility, net of the world-system and status of women; and (4) differences between developing and developed nations in these relationships. Some of these linkages are outlined in Figure 2.2.

(1) The status of women and the structure of income inequality generated by the world-system will have the following effects on fertility (see Figure 2.2). Foreign investment and trade dependency will have a direct positive influence on fertility and an indirect positive influence through heightened income inequality and the declining status of women. Given women's limited resources during underdevelopment, women's labor-force participation and relative share of the labor force should have only a small negative influence on fertility. At the same time, women's share of the three economic sectors should have the following effects: higher participation in agriculture should raise fertility, participation in the service sector will have negligible effects, and, finally, more industrial employment of women should operate to depress fertility. As to the other facets of women's status and fertility, an increase in women's share of tertiary education should lower fertility. Within countries, a longer experience with suffrage, more participation of women in government, and specific legislation for women should have a negative effect on fertility. Last, the number of women's organizations should have a direct negative effect on fertility through the provision of family planning information.

(2) A social setting or health-related variable, infant mortality rate, should be highly related to the extent of world-system intrusion and will be an exogenous intervening mechanism (with the status of women) between the world-system and fertility.

(3) The relative influence of family planning programs on fertility should decline if we incorporate the world-system and the status of women into the model.[12]

(4) Some variations between developed and developing countries can be expected. First, the influence of economic development should enhance the educational and employment opportunities of women and the reduction of fertility in developed countries. At the same time, in developing countries, underdevelopment will not generate the same opportunities or changes in fertility for women as in developing countries.

NOTES

1. An additional example can currently be seen in the United States, where, during a severe recession and high un-

employment of males, the Reagan administration has subtly and not so subtly encouraged a return to women's family roles through public pronouncements, support of antifeminist groups, and elimination of civil rights legislation. At the same time, women's access to abortion and family planning programs has been restricted. Thus, the programs of the "New Right" provide a good example of the manipulation of women's work and reproductive roles in order to regulate the economy. (See Eisenstein 1982 for further analysis of this situation.) Further, this manipulation frequently has been used in the belief that during times of economic crisis, women can drop out of the labor force and their families can rely on women's increased use production or unpaid labor to make up the difference. Unfortunately, as Milkman (1976) notes, services previously produced in the home are increasingly drawn into the market economy; therefore, such services must be purchased, and the capitalist system can no longer rely on relegating women to the home during capitalist crises.

   2. Specific studies of the status of women in Latin America (Youssef 1974; Saffioti 1975, 1977; Nash 1980; Chaney and Schmink 1980; Safa 1981; Shapiro 1980), in the Caribbean (Henry and Wilson 1975; ICRW 1980a, 1980b; Joseph 1980), in Asia (Jahan and Papanek 1979), in Africa (Van Allen 1976; Hafkin and Bay 1976; Matyepse 1977; Lindsay 1980; UNECA 1975), and in the Middle East (Youssef 1974; Mernissi 1977; Allman 1978) have supported this finding.

   3. In Great Britain, only ninety-four women gained posts in Parliament between 1918 and 1971, and only eight women achieved full ministerial rank. The prevailing male authoritarian tradition in the Federal Republic of Germany has limited women's participation to 7.3 percent in the Bundestag (Sanzone 1981). In the United States, there are only two women senators and twenty-four female members of Congress out of 550 congressional positions.

   4. For example, a number of women governors were appointed in the Dominican Republic on the basis that women were less likely to be shot (Newland 1979).

   5. In the United States, the term "sex" was added to the Title VII Amendment of the Civil Rights Act of 1964 in an attempt to defeat the bill. Even in countries with a strong tradition of feminist agitation, such as Great Britain, equal rights legislation has been only recently established (Sanzone 1981).

   6. Semyonov's (1980) analysis is flawed, however, since he did not incorporate measures of the world-system (known to affect income inequality) into his model.

7. More recent historical research has found that although in the long run there was a demographic transition, this transition occurred at different times and in different countries; no common mechanisms that explain the transition have been found (Coale 1973). For example, in some countries, later age at marriage resulted in a decline in fertility, and in still other countries, the increasing usage of contraception led to a fertility decline.

8. Caldwell's analysis is also incomplete because he did not examine the influence of the world-system or the status of women on child-parent cash flows.

9. Davis and Blake (1956) propose that socioeconomic determinants of fertility operate through a set of intermediate mechanisms governing exposure to the risk of fertility, e.g., marriage and contraception. Although specific intermediate mechanisms cannot be directly incorporated into the model, an investigation of the process by which the status of women determines fertility can take place only through a study of these mechanisms. For example, education is assumed to have a direct negative influence on fertility as women gain access to knowledge about contraceptive practices and family limitation and are consequently more apt to limit their fertility (Dixon 1975; Standing 1978). An indirect influence of higher education occurs through later age at marriage and access to labor-force opportunities. Consequently, education operates through these intermediate mechanisms to limit fertility.

There are three reasons why more modern forms of female economic activity have suppressive influences on fertility. First, knowledge and new ideas about family planning, as described in the education section of this chapter, also operate in conjunction with an increased economic motivation to limit fertility. Second, economic activity results in a delay in the age of marriage for younger women, leading to lower fertility over the life cycle (Dixon 1975). Finally, numerous researchers have found that women's labor-force participation can lead to greater power and status within the family (Rosen and Simmons 1971; Piepmeier and Adkins 1973; United Nations 1975; Dixon 1975; Sadik 1974; Tangri 1976). Thus, working women may have a greater voice in fertility and family decision.

10. The relative efficacies of economic development and family planning programs in the reduction of fertility have been debated at great length (see, for example, the proceedings of the 1974 World Population Conference). Some researchers argue that economic development in developing countries is necessary for the reduction of fertility and hence that these countries

should concentrate their meager resources on development efforts, but other researchers argue that population growth is impeding economic development and therefore family planning programs can enhance development efforts. In this research, I assume that both economic development and the reduction of fertility are necessary in developing countries. However, if economic underdevelopment is a consequence of the existing world economic relationships and this form of development leads to higher levels of population growth, researchers and public officials should attempt to maximize their use of limited resources by formulating policies that incorporate the most efficient use of development and family planning programs. Otherwise, family planning programs are likely to be less than effective.

11. Although the process of marginalization occurred also for women in developed countries, these women were gradually brought back into production, and hence a decline in fertility was brought about. The difference for women in developing countries is that under the process of underdevelopment, women may never be brought back in production because of the structural disruption of economies and high male unemployment. Thus, women are relegated to childbearing roles in contrast to women in developed countries.

12. While family planning is depicted and treated as an exogenous variable in this research, the level of economic development, among other variables, is a major determinant of family planning (Hernandez 1981). However, the relationship between development and family planning is not estimated in this research.

This chapter defines the sample, variables, methods, and analysis strategies used to test the hypotheses described in Chapter 2. First, the dependent and independent variables are defined and discussed. Second, measurement issues of data availability and quality for the status-of-women and fertility data are examined. Third, regression equations used in analyzing the status of women and fertility are specified.

SAMPLE

The basic sample for this research consists of 126 nation-states (for lists of specific countries used in analyses see the appendixes). This sample includes state-controlled economies in Eastern Europe but excludes nation-states that have populations less than 250,000 (such as Qatar, United Arab Emirates, Oman, and Bahrain).[1] For countries with populations less than 1 million, some world-system data are unavailable. Thus, the maximum number of cases for which the world-system data can be analyzed is 115.

Nation-state data at the aggregate level are available for the variables of women's educational and economic status for two time points, 1970 (time-1) and 1975. The total fertility rate variable is available for two time points, 1968 (time-1) and 1975.[2] Data for these and other variables are taken from a variety of statistical yearbooks, as cited in the text.

DEPENDENT VARIABLES

The dependent variables relating to women's status consist of economic components. Women's relative share of the total labor force, women's labor-force participation, and women's share of agricultural, industrial, and service sectors constitute separate dependent variables (International Labor Office 1977). Women's shares of the total labor force and of specific sectors are constructed for each country by dividing the total number of adult females in the labor force or sector by the total adult labor force or appropriate sector. In a similar manner, women's labor-force participation rate is calculated by dividing the adult female labor force aged fifteen to sixty-four years by the adult female population.

Fertility is measured by the total fertility rate in each country. This measure represents the average completed family size, or "the number of births 1,000 women would have if they experienced a given set of age-specific birth rates throughout their reproductive span" (Shyrock, Siegel, and Stockwell 1976, p. 314). Since the total fertility rate (TFR) incorporates the actual female childbearing population and age-specific fertility rates, it is a superior measure to other measures of fertility, such as the crude birth rate, which is merely the number of births per total population. Total fertility rate estimates are available from Tsui and Bogue (1978).

INDEPENDENT VARIABLES

Indicators of the world-system and of international and internal or intervening mechanisms are coded from the Zurich Multinational Corporations Project (Ballmer-Cao et al. 1979) unless otherwise specified. This project provides an extensive compilation of world-system and internal nation-state variables. The variables are divided into several groups for analyses: economic development, dependency/investment, intervening mechanisms, and inequality. (See Table 3.1 for a list of variables.) Kilowatt hours per capita (KWH/c) (in logged form) represents a measure of overall economic development. Although several researchers have used the measure of gross national product per capita (GNP/c), kilowatt hours per capita is highly correlated with the GNP/c and is available for more cases.

Dependency variables include indicators of classical dependency or commodity concentration and foreign trade structure. The commodity concentration measure is the value of the most

TABLE 3.1

List of Variables Used

Dependent Variables

Women's share of the labor force
Women's labor force participation rate
Women's share of agriculture
Women's share of industry
Women's share of service
Total fertility rate

Independent Variables

Development Variable:
  Logged kilowatt hours per capita
World-System: Investment/Dependency Variables:
  Commodity concentration
  Foreign trade structure
  Overall foreign investment
  Investment in agriculture
  Investment in manufacturing
  Investment in extraction
  Change in foreign trade
  Change in commodity concentration
  Change in foreign investment
Intervening Variables:
  Size of the labor force
  Change in the size of the labor force
  Size of the service sector
  Bargaining power of labor
  Bureaucratization
  Power sharing with experts
  Urbanization
  State strength
  Social insurance program experience
  Centrally planned economics
  Income inequality (Gini)
Status of Women Control Variables:
  Integration of women into government
  Experience with suffrage
  Women's political status index
  Number of women's groups
  Age at marriage
  Women's share of tertiary educational enrollments
Social Setting/Family Planning Variables:
  Infant mortality rate
  Family planning program effort

---

important export commodity divided by the value of total foreign trade. Foreign trade structure (Galtung 1971) is measured by the composition and diversity of foreign trade in regard to the degree of processing of exports and imports. Thus, the first measure represents the dependency of a nation-state on a certain commodity; the latter measure represents the nation-state's export/import balance of raw materials and processed goods. (See Ballmer-Cao et al. 1979 for further computational details.)

Investment variables include indicators of dependent development or foreign investment: total investment and invest-ment by extractive, agricultural, and manufacturing sectors. The overall foreign investment variable is calculated by dividing the stock of foreign private investments by the square root of kilowatt hours multiplied by population.[3] Specific sectoral foreign investment indicators represent the stock of the sector investment in agriculture, extraction, or manufacturing divided by the square root of kilowatt hours multiplied by population. These variables reflect the levels of investment stocks relative to the size of the population in each country. Ideally, invest-ment data that distinguish between capital- and labor-intensive investment should be used; however, such data are currently unavailable. Additionally, no cross-national manufacturing data exist that separate investment in import substitution plants from that in export-oriented plants. Bornschier and Chase-Dunn (in press), however, note that the former type of manu-facturing investment still constitutes a larger share of all manufacturing investment than export-oriented investment.

The influence of short-term changes in dependency and in investment stocks is represented by residual change scores that are constructed by regressing the level of foreign trade structure, commodity concentration, or foreign investment at time-1 on each variable at time-2.[4] A positive residual score indicates that concentration or investment, for example, has increased at a greater rate than would be expected from earlier trends. A negative residual score indicates a slower-than-expected rate of increase. In analysis these variables are substituted for the original measure at time-2.

Intervening Mechanisms

Intervening mechanisms, which are primarily represented by labor-force variables, are (1) the size of the labor force relative to the population and (2) the tertiary (service) sector as a proportion of the labor force. The overall labor force and the tertiary-sector variables are constructed in a manner similar to the female share variables. The overall labor-force variable is constructed by dividing the adult labor force by the adult population. The tertiary-sector variable is the tertiary labor force divided by the total labor force (International Labor Office [ILO] 1977). An additional measure of change in the size of the labor force is computed by regressing the total labor-force variable in 1970 on the total labor-force measure in 1960, yielding a residualized change score. A positive score means that the size of the labor force relative to the population grew at a faster rate than would be anticipated from an earlier time point.

Other intervening mechanisms are taken from Ballmer-Cao et al. (1979). Bargaining power of labor is measured by the five-year average of the number of workers per industrial dispute. (See Bornschier and Ballmer-Cao 1979 for use of this variable.) No reliable cross-national data exist on union membership. Bureaucratization is the number of clerical workers as a proportion of the nonagricultural labor force. Power sharing with experts is measured by the number of experts per execu- tives and owners outside of agriculture.5 These variables represent the distribution of resources and power within a given nation-state. The indicator of population distribution in urban areas used is urbanization, or the proportion of the population residing in urban areas.

Measures of the state are state strength, social insurance program experience (Ballmer-Cao et al. 1979), and a dummy variable for centrally planned economies. State strength is the amount of government revenues as a percentage of the gross domestic product. Social insurance program experience reflects the years of program experience since 1933. Other measures of social insurance coverage are available, but for significantly fewer cases. In the regression analyses, the state strength variable is used as the major indicator of the influence of the state. The social security program experience variable is used for determining the influence of the state on the value of children. A dummy variable that controls for the effects of centrally planned economies is constructed by assigning a score of 1 to countries with centrally planned economies (eight countries) and 0 to other countries.

Finally, one consequence of world-system relationships is income inequality. This variable is measured by the Gini co- efficient, which is a summary measure of income concentration (Ballmer-Cao et al. 1979). Countries with a high Gini experience greater levels of income inequality. These coefficients are com- puted from household and personal income estimates. Unfortunately, reliable cross-national data on female earnings are unavailable.

Status of Women

Other control variables denoting women's status—women's share of education, political participation, organizational capacity, and proportion of single women—are used in this research. Women's share of tertiary educational enrollments relative to men's is the education control variable, i.e., the number of women in tertiary education divided by total enrollment (UNESCO 1972, 1976).

Indicators of the political status of women or the position of women in government are the following: the integration of women in government or the presence or absence of women at four different levels and sublevels (legislative, judiciary, government, and diplomatic). Dummy variables are coded so that 1 denotes the presence of women and 0 the absence of women at each level and sublevels (thirteen in total). Then the sex variables are summed, yielding a variable with a range of 0 to 13 (United Nations 1970). No information exists, however, on whether these women were appointed or elected and/or what positions they held. The legislative status of women measures include the number of years since suffrage and women's political status index (Boulding et al. 1976; Weiss, Ramirez, and Tracy 1976; Chaney 1979). The suffrage indicator represents the country's experience with suffrage. This variable is constructed by subtracting the date of suffrage from 1970. The general level of women's political rights is represented by a four-point index from Ramirez (1980), by which countries are given points for provisions pertaining to women's equal rights in the constitution, implementation of policies, equal pay legislation, and nation-state endorsement of the United Nations policy of equal rights for women. Although this variable is a more precise measure of women's legislative status than suffrage experience, there may be significant differences among countries on the actual implementation of the policies and provisions in the index (Weiss and Ramirez 1976). The number of known women's groups represents women's organizational capacity and is taken from Hosken (1977). Finally, an indicator of higher age at marriage, which can be affected by legislation and the state, is the proportion of the female population that is single at fifteen to twenty-four years (United Nations 1976; Youssef and Hartley 1979).

Social Setting/Family Planning

A "social setting" or health variable to be used in the determination of fertility is the infant mortality rate, or the number of infant deaths per thousand births (Tsui and Bogue 1978). A measure of family planning program effort is available from Mauldin and Berelson (1978). This measure consists of 30 separate family planning program provisions that are simply summed into a single variable with a range of 0 to 30. (For further information, see Mauldin and Berelson 1978.) This variable, however, is available for only 93 developing countries and no developed countries. Such a data distribution, therefore, may limit the range of variation in the fertility analysis.

MISSING DATA

In cross-national research, missing data are a frequent phenomenon. The data utilized in this analysis are no exception. Data on the dependent variables are available for 126 countries in 1975. Missing data, however, are a greater problem for the independent variables. For the major independent variables, such as kilowatt hours per capita, foreign investments, labor force, and state strength, the average number of cases available is greater than one hundred. When additional variables for analysis are considered, e.g., intervening mechanisms and the status of women, the average number of cases drops below one hundred. Furthermore, the Gini or income inequality variable is available for only seventy-eight cases.

A potential bias from the extent of missing data may result. There might be a bias toward more developed countries that have more highly developed statistical reporting systems and, hence, more complete statistical coverage (Shyrock, Siegel, and Stockwell 1976). Other implications of missing data will be examined more extensively in the analysis section in connection with each set of analyses.

MEASUREMENT ISSUES

Two measurement issues are important for this research: reliability of measures and ratio variables. For research on the status of women, the reliability of national accounts data, e.g., kilowatt hours per capita or gross national product (GNP) per capita, is suspect because income-producing activities of women are not uniformly incorporated into national income accounts (Todaro 1981; International Center for Research on Women [ICRW] 1980a, 1980b; Newland 1980). In some countries, women's water-gathering activities are omitted in the computation of the GNP; in other countries, women's activities may be included, especially if men take some part in that particular activity. Thus, the reliability of the GNP as an indicator of national income and economic development must be questioned. In this research, the kilowatt hours per capita variable is utilized as an indicator of economic development.

Labor-force data on women also have questionable reliability. Frequently, labor-force data are measured differently from country to country, particularly data on the economic activities of women (Boulding et al. 1976; Fong 1973, 1975; Durand 1975; Bose 1979; ICRW 1980a, 1980b). The major measurement problem is the widespread, though uneven, undernumeration of women's work activities. Many countries do not include women's unpaid economic activities in the informal and agricultural sectors in compilations of labor force statistics (Newland 1980; ICRW 1980a, 1980b). The labor-force statistics from the International Labor Office (ILO) (1977) constitute the best cross-national estimates to date in regard to women's unpaid economic contributions. (See Dixon 1982 for another view of these estimates.) Specifically, estimates of women's unpaid labor were incorporated into the ILO's calculation of women's labor-force participation. Dixon (1982), however, notes that women in agriculture are under-represented in these estimates. To the extent that bias remains, the size of regression coefficients should be lowered. The major theoretical relationships formulated in this research propose that foreign investment and dependency affect women's share of the new resources generated by nation-states' incorporation within the world-system. Since my interest is in women's access to the monetarized sector, from which most censuses are taken (ICRW 1980b), these labor-force estimates should provide adequate coverage.

A related issue is the use of separate indicators to represent the status of women. Here theory has proposed four separate dimensions of women's status (educational, economic, political, and organizational), and previous research has found no uniform measures that can be combined into an index (Whyte 1978; Rosaldo 1980). This issue will be addressed in later chapters by first examining the relationships among the status-of-women variables and then examining the specific relationships among investment/dependency, internal mechanisms, and the dimensions represented in the status-of-women variables.

Last, vital statistics are less than reliable because of incomplete statistical reporting or deficient registration systems (Shyrock, Siegel, and Stockwell 1976; Demeny 1979). As a result, I have taken fertility estimates from Tsui and Bogue (1978), who developed estimation techniques that incorporated all available estimates of age-specific fertility rates. For data on infant mortality rates and marital status, the reliability of these measures depends on the completeness of reporting systems and census counts. Census estimates were used, when possible, for measures of marital status. The data on fertility, infant mortality, and marital status should be interpreted with caution.

Ratio Variables

The final measurement issue is the use of ratio variables. These variables may provide a problem in the interpretation of regression estimates because correlated components of the ratios can bias the estimates. Ratio variables are used in this research owing to theoretical concerns (Bollen and Ward 1980; Long 1979). Given the theoretical assumptions of the model, concepts are best expressed as relative proportions of populations and re-sources available for competition (Weiss, Ramirez, and Tracy 1976; Ward and Weiss 1982). In addition, according to theoretical perspectives, the status-of-women concept should be expressed as the status of women relative to men (Dixon 1975; Blumberg 1978). As noted by Long (1979), the use of ratio variables on the basis of theoretical formulations does not necessarily pre-dispose relationships among the ratios in one direction or another.[6] The commonality of components has been kept to a minimum in the construction of variables. Hence, ratio bias should not present any major problems.

METHOD OF ANALYSIS

I have used cross-sectional regression analysis with lagged independent variables to test the hypotheses specified in chapter 2. Regression analysis has been used in a number of world-system studies (see, for example, Bornschier, Chase-Dunn, and Rubinson 1978). In this technique, the analytical focus is on examining how the independent variables influence the range of variation in the dependent variable at one point in time. Thus, the attribution of causality can only be inferred according to theoretical guidelines, and the possibility of reciprocal causation is uncontrolled. As is discussed in chapters 4 and 5, problems with multicollinearity preclude the use of panel regression analysis, which can estimate the effects of the independent variables on changes over time in the dependent variables. In this research, however, the use of independent variables, measured at an earlier time than the dependent variables, should provide better estimates of the influence of the specified independent variables over time than if all variables are measured at the same point in time.

RESEARCH STRATEGY

In this section, the basic structure of analysis will be outlined through the specification of the basic models and statistical techniques. There are two basic equations for analysis. The review of the literature suggests a theoretical rationale for the use of lagged independent variables. As the specified relationships among the world-system (WS), intervening mechanisms (IM), income inequality (IE), the economic status of women (FEM SHA LF), social setting (SS), family planning (FP), and total fertility rate (TFR) take place and change slowly over time, the following assumptions are made: (1) there is a lag effect between the world-system and intervening mechanisms; (2) there is a resulting lag between the intervening mechanisms and the status of women; (3) these lag periods are also appropriate for the determination of fertility. With the available data, the lag period between 1965 (t-2) and 1975 (t) is approximately ten years, or the period of time Kentor (1981) found that investment affected the labor force and urbanization. Further, past research has indicated that women's economic status has long-term effects on women's fertility; fertility has short-term effects on women's economic status (Cramer 1980). Thus, at one time period lag is used between women's economic status and fertility. Given the time constraints on family planning (FP) and the political status of women, these variables will be entered at 1970 (t-1); income inequality will be entered at time-2. Thus, as specified by the following equations, equations 1 and 1a will be used to test hypotheses on the status of women in the labor force. Equations 2 and 2a are for the purpose of testing the fertility hypotheses.

$$\text{FEM SHA LF}_t = \text{IM}_{t-1} + \text{WS}_{t-2} + e \qquad (1)$$

$$\text{FEM SHA LF}_t = \text{IE}_{t-2} + \text{IM}_{t-1} + \text{WS}_{t-2} + e \qquad (1a)$$

$$TFR_t = FEM\ SHA\ LF_{t-1} + FEM\ EDUC_{t-1} +$$
$$WS_{t-2} + SS_{t-1} + FP_{t-1} + e \qquad (2)$$

$$TFR_t = FEM\ SHA\ LF_{t-1} + FEM\ EDUC_{t-1} + IE_{t-2} +$$
$$WS_{t-2} + SS_{t-1} + FP_{t-1} + e \qquad (2a)$$

In the basic regression models, the variables to be used for initial analysis are broken down into several groupings. The status of women as a dependent variable is represented by women's share of the total labor force and the economic sectors, and also by women's labor-force participation rate in 1975. A country's involvement in the world capitalist economy is measured by a variable representing either trade dependency or foreign investment from circa 1967. The level of economic development is indicated by logged kilowatt hours per capita in 1965. Intervening mechanisms are divided into two groups: factors relating to the labor force structure/population distribution and those relating to the state in 1970. In estimating the status-of-women equations, the overall labor-force and state strength variables are used as intervening mechanisms where appropriate. A major control variable for women's economic status is women's share of tertiary education in 1970. Income inequality is measured by the Gini coefficient circa 1967. Owing to data limitations, this variable is entered sequentially into the regression equations. When fertility equations are estimated, another measure of the state that is used is social insurance program experience circa 1970. Finally, the major social setting variable is the infant mortality rate circa 1968. The basic measurement models and equations are specified below.

$$FED\ SHA\ LF_t = FED\ SHA\ LF_{t-1} + FEM\ EDUC_{t-1} +$$
$$TOT\ LF_{t-1} + GOV\ REV_{t-1} + FOR\ DIR\ INV_{t-2} +$$
$$lnKWHC_{t-2} + e \qquad (3)$$

$$FEM\ SHA\ LF_t = FEM\ SHA\ LF_{t-1} + FEM\ EDUC_{t-1} +$$
$$GINI_{t-2} + TOT\ LF_{t-1} + GOV\ REV_{t-1} +$$
$$FOR\ DIR\ INV_{t-2} + lnKWHC_{t-2} + e \qquad (3a)$$

Women's relative share of the labor-force resources (including sectors) is a function of previous levels of economic development (lnKWHC), foreign investment or dependency, state strength (GOV REV), the total labor force (TOT LF), and earlier levels of women's share of tertiary education (FEM EDUC) and income inequality (GINI) for equation 3a. This equation is shown in graphic form in Figure 3.1.

Fertility is determined by previous levels of economic growth, foreign investment or dependency, state strength or social insurance programs (STATE), women's share of the labor force, women's share of tertiary education, infant mortality (INF MORT), and family planning program effort (FAM PLAN) and income inequality in equation 4a. This equation is shown in Figure 3.2.

$$TFR_t = INF\ MORT_{t-1} + FAM\ PLAN_{t-1} +$$
$$FEM\ SHA\ LF_{t-1} + FEM\ EDUC_{t-1} +$$
$$STATE_{t-1} + FOR\ DIR\ INV_{t-2} + lnKWHC_{t-2} + e \qquad (4)$$

$$TFR_t = GINI_{t-2} + INF\ MORT_{t-1} + FAM\ PLAN_{t-1} +$$
$$FEM\ SHA\ LF_{t-1} + STATE_{t-1} + FEM\ EDUC_{t-1} +$$
$$FOR\ DIR\ INV_{t-2} + lnKWHC_{t-2} + e \qquad (4a)$$

Statistical analysis is organized into three parts. First, previous research has suggested that the proposed relationships among investment/dependency, status of women, and fertility differ between developing and developed countries. The possibility of interaction is examined. Interaction terms are

FIGURE 3.1

Diagram of the Economic Status-of-Women Equation

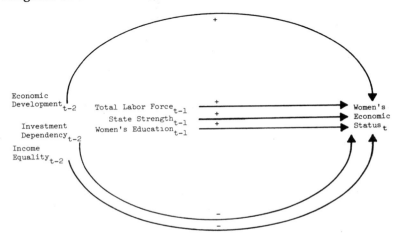

FIGURE 3.2

Diagram of the Fertility Equation

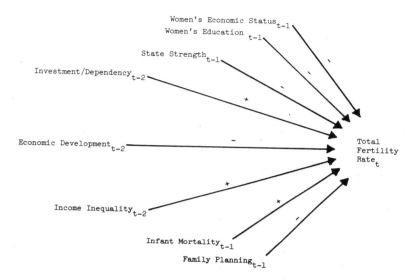

computed by multiplying a world-system indicator by logged kilowatt hours per capita. These terms are then entered into the basic regression equations. If the increment in R^2 in each equation is significant, interaction is controlled for in equations by the inclusion of an interaction term.

Second, the effects of other independent variables are assessed within the basic status-of-women and fertility models. Alternative specifications are estimated where other indicators of investment or dependency—foreign sectoral investment, trade structure, and commodity concentration, or appropriate change scores—are substituted (one at a time owing to a limited number of cases) for the foreign investment variable. Further, other intervening mechanisms, such as tertiary sector, income inequality, bargaining power of labor, bureaucratization, power sharing with experts, and urbanization, are entered into the equations. For the fertility equations, income inequality, infant mortality, and family planning are intervening variables. Other status-of-women variables, representing women's political and organizational status, are added as control variables for the economic status-of-women and fertility equations.

Finally, the issue of specification error arises through the use of income inequality as a determinant of the status of women without the estimation of the reciprocal path. Although previous research has found that, over time, income inequality is a determinant of the status of women (as represented by labor-force participation), I have argued that the status of women can affect the structure of income inequality and that a reciprocal relationship may exist. Since income inequality is available for only one time point and this limitation precludes the estimation of a reciprocal path, specification error is a function of (1) the relationship between the status of women and other determinants of income inequality, and (2) the relationship between the status of women and income inequality. In the analysis that follows, if the latter relationship is high, in the status-of-women equations the coefficient for income inequality is biased upward, especially if the true path is from the status of women to income inequality.

NOTES

1. Additional countries that were excluded are Belize, Brunei, Cape Verde, Cayman Islands, Djibouti, Falkland Islands, Gibraltar, Gilbert Islands, Granada, Liechtenstein, Maldives, Montserrat, Nauru, New Hebrides, Pitcairn, St. Helena, St. Lucia, San Marino, São Tomé, Seychelles, Solomon Islands, Tonga, Turks and Caicos Islands, Tuvalu, Vatican City State, Virgin Islands, West Samoa, and West Indies.

2. Every effort was made to gather data corresponding to the years 1965, 1970, and 1975. Owing to the vagaries of cross-national data, some data were available only for years surrounding these time points. At no time point, however, do data on the dependent variable precede the data on the independent variables.

3. The computation formula for the investment variables is as follows: investment$/\sqrt{(\ln KWHC \times POPULATION)}$. Although population size is the divisor in constructing a number of variables, the different forms of computation for each variable should minimize the problems of correlated error terms that might bias the results. For example, the kilowatt hours measure is logged; the investment variables are computed with the above formula.

4. Time points for the variables used to construct the residual change scores are as follows: foreign trade structure, 1965, 1970; commodity concentration 1965, 1970; foreign investment, 1967, 1973. The sector investment measures are available for only one time point and, thus, change scores are not computed.

5. Power sharing with experts is measured by taking the square root of the product of the number of professional

and technical workers (multiplied by 100) divided by the sum of own-account (self-employed) workers, employers outside agriculture, and administrative and managerial workers (Ballmer-Cao et al. 1979, p. 208).

6. Given the underlying theoretical assumptions of competition between groups for access to resources, the use of ratio variables such as women's share of the labor force and the number of jobs per total population are theoretically essential. Further, theoretical formulations would predict a high relationship between the two variables. But Long (1979) notes that either constant or random measurement error poses problems for substantive interpretation of relationships between ratios. Given the problems of measurement error noted earlier, this topic deserves attention in future research.

4
The Effects of Investment, Dependency, and Intervening Mechanisms on the Economic Status of Women

In chapters 2 and 3, classical dependency and dependent development, represented by measures of investment and dependency, were predicted to reduce women's share of the labor force, economic sectors, and participation rate. The level of economic development, however, was expected to raise women's status. Intervening variables, such as the size of the total labor force and service sector and distributional variables, or bureaucratization, urbanization, and power sharing with experts, were expected to modify the effects of investment and dependency on women's economic status. In contrast, income inequality, one of the consequences of investment and dependency, was predicted to reduce women's status. Finally, variables measuring the educational, organizational, and political status of women were control variables and were expected to enhance women's access to economic resources.

To examine the influence of investment, dependency, and intervening variables on the economic status of women, trends in women's relative share of the labor force, economic sectors, and participation are examined, along with zero-order correlations among independent and dependent variables. A three-part analytical strategy is then utilized. Multivariate analyses are used to assess possible interaction between investment/dependency and development. The additive effects of investment and dependency on women's economic status are estimated. Finally, the effects of other intervening variables, net of investment and dependency, on women's economic status are explored.

DATA AND CORRELATIONS

For 1970 to 1975, changes in women's economic status were minimal. We observe only a slight increase in women's share of the labor force, economic sectors, and participation. For example, women's share of the labor force increased from 29.81 to 30.12 percent. (See Table 4.1 for means, standard deviations, and correlations, and Appendix A for the countries used in analysis.)[1] For this sample of nation-states, women's average share of the labor force, measured by women as a proportion of the total labor force, was 30 percent. Women's participation rate was 40 percent. Considerable cross-national variation existed in women's share of the labor force and participation rates. For example, women's share of the labor force in 1975 varied from 4 to 50 percent; women's participation rate varied even more widely, from 3 to 87 percent. Women's share of economic sectors during the same period was somewhat lower. In 1975, women were only 20 percent of the workers in the industrial sector, 26 percent of the agricultural sector, and 34 percent of the service sector. Thus, women constituted a substantial proportion of the world's labor force but were unequally represented in the overall labor force across countries and across economic sectors.

Investment and Dependency Variables

Examination of the zero-order relationships in Table 4.1 confirms the theoretical expectations of negative relationships between investment/dependency variables and the status of women. In general, investment and dependency are negatively correlated with women's economic status in 1975. Foreign investment and trade dependency, as represented by commodity concentration and foreign and sector (or transnational) investment indicators, have fairly consistent and moderate negative correlations with the status-of-women indicators. The only deviations from this pattern are found for transnational (TNC) investments in agriculture and manufacturing, which have small and positive correlations with the women's labor-force indicators (except with women's share of industry). The foreign trade structure variable also has a stronger positive correlation with women's economic status. This latter relationship is reasonable because more diverse trade structures should be related to higher economic status for women.

The economic development variable has low negative correlations with most of the economic status-of-women variables. The

TABLE 4.1

Number of Cases, Means, Standard Deviations, and Correlations

Varia-bles	PWLF	WLFP	PWAG	PWSER	PWIND	KWHC	KWH2	TRSTR	CMCON	FDI	MNCAG	MNCEX	MNCM	ΔTRS	ΔCOM	ΔFDI	DCPE	GINI	TLF
N	126	126	126	126	126	126	126	104	87	114	114	114	114	104	79	115	126	75	126
$\bar{X}$	30.12	40.70	33.64	26.50	20.28	5.72	40.50D-5	-.379	43.43	54.97	7.55	24.00	16.40	-1.32E-16	5.49E-15	3.10E-14	.06	44.71	64.30
Sd	11.97	21.20	15.74	17.27	12.58	1.76	10.78D-6	.33	22.95	43.28	16.03	35.22	15.50	.08	9.29	26.97	.24	10.26	11.53
PWLF	1.00																		
WLFP	.974	1.00																	
PWAG	.493	.388	1.00																
PWSER	.823	.831	.081	1.00															
PWIND	.548	.537	-.459	.331	1.00														
KWHC	-.011	-.122	-.408	-.181	-.012	1.00													
KWH2	.196	.148	.356	-.047	.105	.565	1.00												
TRSTR	.216	.170	.209	.191	.249	.498	.381	1.00											
CMCON	-.282	-.214	-.310	-.197	-.137	.463	-.345	-.641	1.00										
FDI	-.222	-.216	-.035	-.028	-.260	-.012	-.076	-.382	.506	1.00									
MNCAG	.030	-.042	-.119	-.229	-.169	-.185	-.162	-.276	.221	.753	1.00								
MNCEX	-.251	-.236	.098	-.153	-.260	-.064	-.151	-.370	.548	.140	.316	1.00							
MNCM	.056	.019	-.098	.101	-.225	.174	.128	-.114	-.121	-.138	.324	.157	1.00						
ΔTRS	-.207	-.209	-.141	-.159	-.273	.052	.017	-.000	.000	.140	-.079	-.134	-.016	1.00					
ΔCOM	-.038	-.045	-.067	-.273	-.253	-.019	.014	-.038	-.173	-.000	-.165	-.248	-.137	-.124	1.00				
ΔFDI	.217	.171	.267	.158	.158	.308	.226	.375	.000	-.350	-.130	-.154	-.228	.014	-.074	1.00			
DCPE	.300	.286	.263	.253	.308	.295	.214	.280	-.367	.436	-.180	-.188	-.292	-.163	.010	-.030	1.00		
GINI	-.289	-.269	-.210	-.360	-.401	-.267	-.374	-.499	-.214	.255	-.165	-.211	-.156	-.118	.106	-.270	-.555	1.00	
TLF	.923	.975	.286	.489	.575	-.034	.182	.071	-.425	-.180	.114	-.141	.044	-.212	-.062	.137	.206	-.161	1.00
ΔTLF	.198	.184	.260	.129	.314	-.267	.433	.331	-.323	.007	-.033	-.141	.186	.019	-.073	.392	.187	-.360	.172
SEVLF	-.163	-.286	-.430	.014	.014	.789	.465	.377	-.331	.113	.007	-.008	.273	.023	-.104	.301	-.023	-.299	-.424
GGR	-.049	.112	-.167	-.140	.702	.702	.428	.398	-.261	.084	-.205	.010	.125	-.048	.162	.221	-.054	-.405	-.200
BUREAU	.250	.232	.253	-.080	.561	.561	.449	.557	-.574	-.062	-.161	-.367	.264	.124	.046	-.384	-.023	-.444	.197
STRIKE	.004	-.030	-.072	-.012	.145	.145	.023	.128	-.110	-.033	-.050	-.123	.174	.086	-.056	-.003	.000	-.222	-.052
URBPOP	-.091	-.187	.320	.036	.807	.807	.432	.454	-.356	-.016	-.240	-.147	.208	.070	-.055	.281	.129	-.323	-.323
POWER	.496	.489	.577	.334	.575	-.575	.343	-.406	-.359	-.263	-.156	-.276	-.101	-.226	.175	.281	.752	-.644	.378
LPWLF	.999	.976	.478	.577	.545	-.034	.182	.204	-.270	-.221	.037	-.242	-.044	-.212	-.031	.209	.298	-.275	.929
LWLFP	.968	.998	.834	.834	.528	-.161	.120	.139	-.188	-.205	-.221	.016	.016	-.216	-.040	.156	.266	-.230	.983
LPWAG	.833	.840	.999	.346	.346	-.185	-.047	.187	-.195	-.303	.029	-.224	-.154	-.146	.102	.070	.316	-.231	.817

(continued)

Table 4.1 (continued)

Varia-bles	PWLF	WLFP	PWSER	PWAG	PWIND	KWHC	KWH2	TRSTR	CMCON	FDI	MNCAG	MNCEX	MNCM	△ TRS	△ COM	△ FDI	DCPE	GINI	TLF
N	126	126	126	126	126	126	126	104	87	114	114	114	114	104	79	115	126	75	126
X̄	30.12	40.70	33.64	26.50	20.28	5.72	40.50D-5	-.379	43.23	54.97	7.55	24.00	16.40	-1.32E-16	5.49E-15	3.10E-14	.06	44.71	64.30
Sd.	11.97	21.20	15.74	17.27	12.58	1.76	10.78D-6	.33	22.95	43.28	16.03	35.22	15.50	.08	9.29	26.97	.24	10.26	11.53
LPWSER	.387	.479	.999	.058	.463	.388	.309	.195	-.294	-.031	-.026	-.109	.101	-.100	-.068	.265	.245	-.189	.281
LPWIND	.523	.536	.474	.304	.999	-.012	.099	.236	-.129	-.322	-.162	-.248	-.218	-.160	-.277	.155	.247	-.335	.476
LPF3ED	-.076	.018	.409	-.156	.137	.613	.307	.297	-.274	-.171	-.061	-.176	.025	-.010	-.214	.166	.324	-.469	-.185
WGPS	-.009	.061	-.249	-.094	.046	.391	.615	.419	-.314	-.187	-.205	-.183	-.066	-.045	.066	.123	-.127	-.047	-.055
SUFFEX	.129	.204	.405	-.024	.141	.613	.460	.298	-.360	-.194	.161	-.313	.180	.077	-.139	.287	.177	-.471	-.036
WGVINT	-.032	.016	.293	-.186	.116	.508	.349	.360	-.301	-.115	.058	-.204	.079	.101	-.124	-.236	.149	-.311	-.100
POLINX	.016	-.002	.065	.033	.180	.154	.012	.233	-.047	-.295	-.027	-.213	-.213	.163	-.213	.055	-.453	-.247	-.025
PSW1524	.046	.136	.506	-.076	.326	.539	.190	.466	-.500	.113	-.155	-.245	.334	.100	-.029	.425	.058	.295	-.066

Varia-bles	△ TLF	SEVLF	GGR	BUREAU	STRIKE	URBPOP	POWER	LPWLF	LWLFP	LPWAG	LPWSER	LPWIND	LPF3ED	WGPS	SUFFEX	WGVINT	POLINX	PSW1524
N	126	126	117	54	62	122	49	126	126	126	126	126	115	95	109	78	126	74
X̄	6.20E-15	29.10	21.77	11.87	460.87	39.43	8.80	29.81	40.52	26.41	33.10	20.16	27.96	3.99	23.43	5.94	1.25	62.41
Sd.	1.98	15.78	9.19	4.16	610.93	23.98	4.91	12.28	21.71	17.35	15.83	12.69	12.62	3.47	15.97	2.73	1.15	14.93

PWLF
WLFP
PWAG
PWSER
PWIND
KWHC
KWH2
TRSTR
CMCON
FDI
MNCAG
MNCEX

	TLF	Δ TLF	SEVLF	GGR	BUREAU	STRIKE	URBPOP	POWER	LPWLF	LWLFP	LPWAG	LPWSER	LPWIND	LPF3ED	WGPS	SUFFEX	WGVINT	POLINX	PSW1524
MNCM																			
Δ TRS																			
Δ COM																			
Δ FDI																			
DCPE																			
GINI																			
TLF	1.00																		
Δ TLF	.252	1.00																	
SEVLF	.198	.580	1.00																
GGR	.487	.532	.479	1.00															
BUREAU	.532	.174	-.071	.094	1.00														
STRIKE	.065	.832	.565	.496	.234	1.00													
URBPOP	.265	.161	.740	.191	-.154	.184	1.00												
POWER	.441	-.187	-.062	.233	-.004	-.116	.184	1.00											
LPWLF	.192	-.319	-.136	.194	.005	-.222	-.039	.484	1.00										
LWLFP	.162	-.430	-.169	.005	-.076	-.303	.309	.453	.972	1.00									
LPWAG	.008	.025	-.173	-.246	.065	.309	-.036	.237	.841	.843	1.00								
LPWSER	.263	.530	-.144	-.096	-.014	.519	.173	.561	.467	.533	.515	1.00							
LPWIND	.129	.345	.302	-.174	.173	.237	.043	.464	.320	.336	.355	.479	1.00						
LPF3ED	.140	.532	.316	.174	.173	.546	.237	.179	-.154	-.096	-.077	-.106	.141	1.00					
WGPS	.158	.316	.345	.235	.043	.316	.043	.237	.246	.044	.000	.396	.044	.254	1.00				
SUFFEX	.272	.549	.350	.329	.235	.549	.184	.546	.394	.139	-.022	.246	.139	.486	.317	1.00			
WGVINT	.087	.350	-.439	-.051	.164	.350	.151	.434	.293	.126	-.056	.394	.126	.500	.369	.418	1.00		
POLINX	-.035	-.057	.028	-.051	.164	.028	.164	.132	.063	.181	-.003	.063	.181	.222	-.023	.077	.270	1.00	
PSW1524	.215	.645	.375	.303	.161	.603	.181	.109	.013	-.076	.109	.506	.322	.489	.105	.308	.251	-.013	1.00

Variable definitions (terms in parentheses are used in regression tables)

PWLF	women's share of the labor force, 1975 (FEM SHA LF)
WLFP	women's labor force participation rate, 1975 (FEM LFP)
PWSER	women's share of the service sector, 1975 (FEM SHA SERV)
PWAG	women's share of the agricultural sector, 1975 (FEM SHA AG)
PWIND	women's share of the industrial sector, 1975 (FEM SHA IND)
KWHC	logged kilowatt hours per capita, 1965
KWH2	logged kilowatt hours per capita (squared), 1965
TRSTR	foreign trade structure, 1965 (FOR TRA STR)
CMCON	commodity concentration, 1965 (COM CONC)
FDI	foreign investment, 1967 (FOR DIR INV)
MNCAG	multinational (MNC) investment in agriculture, 1967 (MNC INV AG)
MNCEX	MNC investment in extraction, 1967 (MNC INV EX)

(continued)

Table 4.1 (continued)

MNCM	MNC investment in manufacturing, 1967 (MNC INV MAN)
Δ TRS	residual change score foreign trade structure, 1965-70 (Δ FOR TRA STR)
Δ COM	residual change score commodity concentration, 1965-70 (Δ COM CONC)
Δ FDI	residual change score foreign investment, 1967-1973 (Δ FOR DIR INV)
DCPE	centrally planned economies
GINI	income inequality, circa 1967
TLF	total labor force relative to adult population, 1970 (TOT LF)
Δ TLF	residual change score total labor force, 1960-70 (Δ TOT LF)
SEVLF	service labor force relative to total labor force (SERV LF)
GGR	government revenues as a percent of the gross domestic product, 1970 (GOV REV)
BUREAU	bureaucratization, 1970
STRIKE	average number of strikes, 1970
URBPOP	proportion of the population in urban areas, 1970
POWER	power sharing with experts, 1970
LPWLF	lagged women's share of the labor force, 1970
LWLFP	lagged women's labor force participation rate, 1970
LPWAG	lagged women's share of the agricultural sector, 1970
LPWSER	lagged women's share of the service sector, 1970
LPWIND	lagged women's share of the industrial sector, 1970
LPF3ED	lagged women's share of tertiary education, 1970 (FEM TERT ED)
WGPS	number of women's groups (WOM GPS)
SUFFEX	years experience with suffrage, 1970 (SUFF EXP)
WGVINT	integration of women in levels of government, 1970 (WOM GOV)
POLINX	political rights index (POL RTS)
PSW1524	proportion of single women aged 15-24, 1970 (% SING WOM)

correlation of this variable, however, with women's share of the service sector is larger and positive (r = .38). Scatter plots show that the other negative relationships of economic development with the status of women suggest a curvilinear relationship between measures of economic development and the economic status of women. Women's economic status is higher at the lower and upper levels of economic development. These curvilinear relationships are examined further in regression analysis.

Intervening and Control Variables

The major intervening variable in the determination of women's status is the size of the labor force. Other intervening and control variables are size of the service sector relative to the adult labor force, state strength, income inequality, bureaucratization, power sharing with experts, and other status-of-women variables. As expected, the size of the total labor force in 1970 has strong positive relationships with the women's labor-force indicators (see Table 4.1). The residual change variable for the total labor force from 1960 to 1970 has smaller but positive relationships with these same indicators. In contradiction with the argument that the expansion of the service sector is uniformly related to the expansion of women's economic opportunities, the size of the service sector in 1970 has moderately negative correlations with the economic status indicators. Likewise, both state strength and income inequality are negatively related to women's economic status, with the exception of the positive correlation of state strength with women's share of the service sector. The negative correlations of state strength with women's share of economic resources and participation are unexpected, given other research that indicates positive relationships (Weiss, Ramirez, and Tracy 1976). The negative correlation of income inequality with women's economic status is consistent with the interpretation that the status of women reflects the level of inequality in a nation-state.

Additional intervening mechanisms vary in the strength of their relationships with the economic status-of-women variables. Power sharing with experts represents equality and is positively correlated with women's share of the labor force in the agricultural, industrial, and service sectors and with participation rates. Bureaucratization has a similar pattern of relationships, but with smaller zero-order correlations. Urbanization has a positive relationship with women's share of the service sector, but correlates negatively with women's participation and women's share of agriculture. Finally, the union or strike indicator has a negligible relationship with all economic status of women indicators—contrary to the predicted relationships.

Status-of-Women Control Variables

The major status-of-women control or intervening variable is women's share of tertiary education. The number of women's groups, experience with suffrage, integration of women in government, and women's political rights are additional control variables. Women's share of tertiary education in 1970 is related to some indicators of women's economic status, but not to others. For example, women's education share is positively correlated with women's share of the service and industrial sectors, while this same education variable has a negligible relationship with women's overall share of the labor force. Women's education is negatively correlated with women's labor-force participation and share of agriculture. Because of the historically positive relationships between education and women's share of the labor force and participation rates in developed countries, the negligible or negative relationships are unexpected. These relationships could indicate that, cross-nationally and over time, education has different effects on women's share of economic resources. The relationship between women's education and economic status also might vary, depending on which economic status indicator is used. As to the other status-of-women variables, there is a general pattern of positive relationships between these variables and the economic status-of-women variables. Experience with suffrage is moderately and positively correlated with women's economic status. Of the economic indicators, women's share of service sector exhibits the most consistent positive relationships with the other status-of-women variables. However, for these other variables, the relationships with women's economic status are frequently small or negligible.

Thus, examination of the zero-order correlations produces moderate support for the hypothesized relationships. The empirical relationships among the investment, dependency, and economic status-of-women variables, however, need to be analyzed in a multivariate context. The next few sections report the results of regression analyses, which were organized into three steps. First, tests of interaction effects between investment/dependency and development on women's economic status were performed. Second, if no interaction effects were found, the additive effects of investment and dependency on women's share of the labor force, participation rate, and economic sectors were estimated, controlling for economic development, the total labor force, and women's share of tertiary education.[2] Finally, the relative effects of alternative intervening and control variables were evaluated by including these variables separately in the basic regression model.

EFFECTS OF INVESTMENT AND DEPENDENCY

Women's Share of the Labor Force and Participation

As the first analysis step, the possibility of interaction between dependency/investment and level of economic development (measured by kilowatt hours per capita) was tested by constructing interaction terms with separate dependency/investment indicators and logged kilowatt hours per capita. No significant interaction effects were found by controlling for level of development, change in the total labor force, and women's share of tertiary education.[3]

Tables 4.2 and 4.3 present the results of the basic model, that is, regressing the economic status of women, as represented by women's labor-force share and participation, on separate dependency and investment indicators while controlling for KWH/c, change in the total labor force, and women's share of education. A different dependency or investment indicator is included in each equation (column). The indicators of classical dependency are significant in these equations. The diversity of a country's foreign trade structure has a positive effect on women's economic status, in contrast with the negative effect of commodity concentration. Of the dependent development or investment indicators, only overall foreign investment and multinational investment in extraction are significant, and these forms of investment operate to depress women's share of the labor force and participation. As can be seen by the differences between the unstandardized coefficients in the two tables, dependency and investment variables have a stronger impact on women's participation than on women's share.

At the same time, higher levels of economic development reduce women's share and participation. A test for curvilinear relationships between development and women's economic status, performed by adding a squared development term to the equations, is not significant. As to the effects of the major intervening and control variables, the change in the labor force is

TABLE 4.2

Ordinary Least Squares (OLS) Estimates of the Influence of Investment and Dependency on Women's Share of the Labor Force, 1975

Variables	Unstandardized and Standardized Coefficients					
	Women's Share					
FOR TRA STR[a]	8.15^b					
	(.25)					
COM CONC[a]		$-.13^b$				
		(-.24)				
FOR DIR INV[a]			$-.05^c$			
			(-.18)			
MNC INV EX[a]				$-.07^b$		
				(-.20)		
ΔFOR TRA STR[a] (65-70)					-28.87^b	
					(-.20)	
ΔFOR DIR INV (67-73)						$.10^b$
						(.24)
KWHC[a]	-2.52^b	-1.88^c	$-.99$	$-.97$	-1.69^c	-1.90^b
	(-.38)	(-.27)	(-.14)	(-.14)	(-.26)	(-.28)
FEM TERT ED[d]	.10	.11	.04	.04	.09	-.01
	(.11)	(.11)	(.04)	(.04)	(.09)	(-.01)
ΔTOT LF[d] (60-70)	1.25^b	1.24^c	1.59^b	1.41^b	1.60^b	.97
	(.23)	(.22)	(.27)	(.24)	(.29)	(.16)
Intercept	46.06	42.02	37.67	36.44	38.50	40.48
R^2 (explained variance)	.13	.11	.10	.10	.13	.13
N (number of cases)	95	83	105	105	95	97

[a]Measured at t-2, or circa 1965.
[b]$p < .05$.
[c]$p < .10$.
[d]Measured at t-1, or circa 1970.
Note: Variables are defined in Table 4.1. Standardized regression coefficients are in parentheses.

TABLE 4.3

OLS Estimates of the Influence of Investment and Dependency on Women's Labor-Force Participation Rate, 1975

Variables	Unstandardized and Standardized Coefficients					
	Women's Participation Rate					
FOR TRA STR[a]	15.78[b] (.27)					
COM CONC[a]		-.19[c] (-.21)				
FOR DIR INV[a]			.10[b] (-.20)			
MNC INV EX[a]				-.13[b] (-.21)		
ΔFOR TRA STR[a] 65-70					-50.69[b] (.20)	
ΔFOR DIR INV[a] 67-73						.16[b] (.22)
KWHC[a]	-5.65[b] (.49)	-3.92[b] (-.33)	-2.65[b] (-.22)	-2.61[b] (-.22)	-4.08[b] (-.35)	-4.31[b] (-.36)
FEM TERT ED[d]	.09 (.05)	.07 (.04)	-.03 (-.02)	-.03 (-.01)	.06 (.04)	-.14 (-.08)
ΔTOT LF[d] 60-70	2.41 (.25)	2.36[b] (.24)	2.93[b] (.28)	2.60[b] (.25)	3.07[b] (.31)	1.90[c] (.18)
Intercept	78.46	66.93	62.72	60.3	63.95	67.54
R^2	.19	.12	.13	.13	.18	.18
N	95	82	105	105	95	97

[a]Measured at t-2, or circa 1965.
[b]$\underline{p} < .05$.
[c]$\underline{p} < .10$.
[d]Measured at t-1, or circa 1970.
Note: Variables are defined in Table 4.1. Standardized regression coefficients are in parentheses.

related to higher economic status for women. Women's share of education is nonsignificant. Thus, the most important determinants of women's share of the labor force are the relatively equal effects of investment/dependency, the change in the labor force, and KWH/c. Women's labor-force participation is most strongly determined by KWH/c, followed by the size of the labor force and investment and dependency.

Finally, in analyses not reported here, the size of the service sector was found to have a negative influence on women's share of the labor force and participation (Ward 1982). The expansion of the service sector leads to a reduction in women's share of the labor force, except in the case of the commodity concentration equation, where the effects of the service sector are nonsignificant. Additionally, in other equations, foreign investment becomes nonsignificant when the size of the service sector is controlled. These results suggest that the excessive growth of service sector discussed by Evans and Timberlake (1980) has some negative economic consequences for women and possibly serves as an intervening mechanism in determining their status.

An additional dimension of investment and dependency is the influence of short-term changes in the diversity of foreign trade, commodity concentration, and foreign investment on women's share of the labor force and participation. Of the three residual change variables,[4] the effect of the change in trade structure diversity is significant and negative. The change in foreign investment has a significant and positive effect. Thus, although the level of foreign trade structure at time-2 has a positive influence on women's share of the labor force and participation, when the diversity of foreign trade structures is incorporated, this new variable operates in accordance with the predictions drawn from Galtung's argument (1971). Less diverse trade structures result in less economic growth and, hence, a lesser share for women of economic resources.

The upward growth in foreign investment or short-term flows has a positive influence on women's share and participation. Other research suggests that such a result indicates only a short-run trend in women's employment, in contrast with the long-run negative effects of unstable foreign investment (NACLA 1977; Grossman 1978/79; Ehrenreich and Fuentes 1981; Elson and Pearson 1981b). However, given the overall negative effects of foreign investment through transnational corporations, less diverse trade structures, and commodity concentration, the short-run positive effects of foreign investment may well be counteracted by the long-run deleterious effects of investment and dependency on developing nations.

These results, however, could be spurious because of the inclusion of centrally planned economies in the sample.[5] These nation-states record low levels of Western foreign investment, are uniquely located within the world-system as semiperipheral nation-states that compete with core nations for the resources of the periphery, and have additional provisions for incorporating women in the labor force (Wallerstein 1974, 1979; Lapidus 1978). Thus, the negative effects of investment and dependency found in Tables 4.2 and 4.3 could be related to mixing the effects of centrally planned economies with the effects of investment.

To test this possibility, as I mentioned in Chapter 3, a dummy variable for centrally planned economies is constructed by assigning a score of 1 to countries with centrally planned economies (eight Eastern European countries) and 0 to other countries. Then the regression equations are reestimated. The results for women's share of the labor force are presented in Table 4.4. Some changes in the size and significance of the regression coefficients are apparent. Foreign investment and transnational (TNC) investment in extraction become nonsignificant in the women's share equations. Foreign investment and change in the trade structure become nonsignificant in the participation equations (Ward 1982). Concurrently, the coefficient for TNC investment in manufacturing becomes positive and significant, suggesting a suppressor effect. The effects of state efforts to incorporate women into the economy are large, as is indicated by the unstandardized regression coefficients of the centrally planned economy dummy variable. Women's share of the labor force increases in the range of 11 to 19 percent, while women's participation increases by 20 to 35 percent in centrally planned economies.[6]

These results are interesting in that they contrast two potential types of dependency and investment, Western and centrally planned. For example, when the sample is taken as a whole, foreign investment and dependency have significant negative effects because of the inclusion of centrally planned economies that have low levels of Western investment and high economic status of women. In countries with high levels of Western investment, however, women tend to have lower economic status. The argument could be made that the nature of Western capitalist investment and the pursuant marginalization of women from the labor force is one of the major factors that leads to a decline in the economic status of women. Centrally planned investment and economies appear to utilize women workers more fully than those countries influenced by Western investment, which, until recently, have limited the entrance

TABLE 4.4

OLS Estimates of the Influence of Investment, Dependency, and State-Controlled Economies on Women's Share of the Labor Force, 1975

Variables	Unstandardized and Standardized Coefficients				
	Women's Share				
FOR TRA STR[a]	6.61^b				
	$(.20)$				
FOR DIR INV[a]		$-.02$			
		$(-.08)$			
MNC INV EX[a]			$-.05$		
			$(-.15)$		
MNC INV MAN[a]				$.15^b$	
				$(.19)$	
ΔFOR TRA STR[a]					-23.01^b
					$(-.16)$
CENT PLAN ECON	12.84^c	14.21^c	14.47^c	19.04^c	12.87^c
	$(.23)$	$(.32)$	$(.32)$	$(.42)$	$(.23)$
KWHC[a]	-2.56^c	1.36	-1.27	-1.82^c	-1.89^c
	$(-.39)$	$(-.20)$	$(.19)$	$(.27)$	$(.29)$
FEM TERT ED[d]	$.06$	$-.01$	$-.03$	$.01$	$.05$
	$(.07)$	$(-.01)$	$(-.03)$	$(.01)$	$(.06)$
ΔTOT LF[d]	1.21^c	1.39^c	1.24^c	1.20^c	1.49
	$(.22)$	$(.24)$	$(.21)$	$(.20)$	$(.27)$
Intercept	46.21	38.53	38.64	36.81	40.10
R^2	.18	.18	.19	.20	.18
N	95	105	105	105	95

[a]Measured at t-2, or circa 1965.
[b]$p < .10$.
[c]$p < .05$.
[d]Measured at t-1, or circa 1970.
Note: Variables are defined in Table 4.1. Standardized regression coefficients are in parentheses.

of women into the labor force. These results raise an additional
issue: the potentially negative effects on the economic status
of women that arise from the introduction of Western investment
into centrally planned economies.

Women's Share of Economic Sectors

Less aggregated measures of women's economic status or
women's share of specific sectors are also related to measures
of investment and dependency (see Tables 4.5 and 4.6). Greater
diversity of foreign trade structure has a significant and positive
influence on women's share of industrial and agricultural sectors,
while heightened commodity concentration has a negative influence only on women's share of agriculture. Overall foreign
investment operates to lower women's share of industrial and
agricultural jobs. In these same sectors, TNC investment in
manufacturing decreases women's share. Further, TNC investment in agriculture has a negative influence on women's share
of the industrial sector. Of the three changes in dependency
and investment variables, only the change in commodity concentration variable has a significant influence on women's share
of industry and agriculture. This variable lowers women's
share of industry and raises women's share of agriculture.
Investment and dependency variables have little effect on women's
share of the service sector. The determinants of women's share
of the service sector are discussed in a later section.
In the industrial and agricultural equations, the effects
of the intervening or control variables differ across sectors.
KWH/c becomes unstable across all the regression equations.
Although the size of the labor force in 1970 is consistently
significant in these equations, women's share of education has
a positive and significant influence only on women's share of
industry.[7] Hence, the strongest effects for women's share of
industry are observed for the size of the labor force, investment/
dependency, and education. The most important variables for
women's share of agriculture are size of the labor force and
investment/dependency.
The effects of centrally planned economies on these results
is also of interest. When entered into the women's share of
industry equations, the dummy variable representing centrally
planned economies is nonsignificant. The results of these
equations are not reported in detail. This dummy variable is
significant, however, in the women's share of agriculture
equations; but, in contrast to earlier findings, the investment

TABLE 4.5

OLS Estimates of the Influence of Investment and Dependency on Women's Share of the Industrial Sector, 1975

Variables	Unstandardized and Standardized Coefficients				
	Women's Industrial Share				
FOR TRA STR[a]	8.56[b] (.23)				
FOR DIR INV[a]		-.06[b] (-.20)			
MNC INV AG[a]			-.21[b] (-.23)		
MNC INV MAN[a]				-.18[b] (-.23)	
ΔCOM CONC[d] 65-70					-.25[c] (-.20)
KWHC[a]	-2.07[b] (-.28)	-.32 (-.04)	-.82 (-.11)	-.01 (-.00)	-.96 (-.14)
FEM TERT ED[d]	.34[b] (.33)	.22[b] (.22)	.30[b] (.30)	.25[b] (.25)	.28[b] (.28)
TOT LF[d]	.49[b] (.43)	.51[b] (.47)	.57[b] (.52)	.57[b] (.52)	.49[b] (.45)
Intercept	-3.76	-12.57	-17.66	-19.06	-12.37
R^2	.31	.32	.33	.33	.32
N	95	105	105	105	75

[a]Measured at t-2, or circa 1965.
[b]$p < .05$.
[c]$p < .10$.
[d]Measured at t-1, or circa 1970.
Note: Variables are defined in Table 4.1. Standardized regression coefficients are in parentheses.

TABLE 4.6

OLS Estimates of the Influence of Investment and Dependency on Women's Share of the Agricultural Sector, 1975

Variables	Unstandardized and Standardized Coefficients				
	Women's Agricultural Share				
FOR TRA STR[a]	10.64[b] (.22)				
COM CONC[a]		-.10[c] (-.13)			
FOR DIR INV[a]			-.07[b] (-.17)		
MNC INV MAN[a]				-.23[b] (-.20)	
ΔCOM CONC[d] 65-70					.25[c] (.14)
KWHC[a]	-1.27 (-.13)	-.08 (-.01)	.89 (.09)	1.28[c] (.13)	.38 (.04)
FEM TERT ED[d]	-.06 (-.04)	-.17 (-.12)	-.15 (-.10)	-.12 (-.08)	-.09 (-.07)
TOT LF[d]	1.06[c] (.71)	1.16[b] (.76)	1.18[b] (.78)	1.26[b] (.83)	1.20[b] (.79)
Intercept	-29.16	-40.24	-47.37	-55.16	-51.54
R^2	.64	.64	.68	.69	.64
N	95	83	105	105	75

[a] Measured at t-2, or circa 1965.
[b] $p < .05$.
[c] $p < .10$.
[d] Measured at t-1, or circa 1970.

Note: Variables are defined in Table 4.1. Standardized regression coefficients are in parentheses.

and dependency variables remain significant, albeit smaller in size. The influence of centrally planned economies on women's share of agriculture is also apparent: Women's share increases in a range of 9 to 11 percent (Ward 1982). Hence, centrally planned economies have a significant net influence on women's share of agriculture but nonsignificant effects on women's share of industry.

Thus, classical dependency and foreign investment, net of the level of development and the size of the labor force, operate to reduce women's share of economic resources relative to men's, in particular, women's share of specific economic sectors. These latter results persist for women's industrial- and agricultural-sector shares, even after controlling for the effects of centrally planned economies. As to future implications, some investment and dependency indicators do provide short-run increments to women's overall employment. In the long run, these factors and the material consequences of under-development should eventually lower women's economic status. The employment of women generated by foreign and manufacturing investment is frequently minimal and/or unstable in the global economy, owing to TNCs' utilizing capital-intensive facilities and seeking continued profits. More specifically, foreign investment and TNC investment in manufacturing have direct negative effects on women's share of industry, despite the purported benefits of such investments.

OTHER INTERVENING MECHANISMS

As noted earlier, a number of intervening and control variables, e.g., income inequality, state strength, distributional factors, and the organizational and political status of women, are expected to mediate the effects of investment and dependency on the economic status of women. These variables are included separately in the basic regression equations to evaluate their effects, net of investment and dependency on women's share of the labor force and industrial and agricultural sectors.[8] Results are reported in the next two sections.

Women's Share of the Labor Force

Income inequality is predicted to lower women's relative share of economic resources. The performance of this variable is inconsistent, and these results must be treated with caution

because of the reduced number of cases. The influence of
income inequality is generally nonsignificant, with the exception
of the equations for foreign investment and TNC investment in
extraction. In these equations this measure has a significant
negative influence, and the effects of the investment variables
are reduced to nonsignificance. The TNC investment in extraction equation is shown in Table 4.7 (first column). Furthermore,
when the state-controlled economy dummy variable is entered
into the equation, the income inequality measure is no longer
significant. [9] The general pattern of results for income inequality,
however, suggests negative but nonsignificant effects for the
remaining equations. Hence, income inequality has an unstable
but negative influence on women's share of the labor force.
This finding contradicts Semyonov's (1980) findings of strong
negative effects of income inequality, but his research omitted
measures of investment and dependency.

Other researchers have reported that the strength of the
state has operated to increase women's share of the labor force
(Weiss, Ramirez, and Tracy 1976). Yet, in separate analyses
not reported here (Ward 1982), the state was found to have,
at the most, a small negative influence. (These analyses did
not control for the level of economic development because of
multicollinearity.) Further, this influence was unstable and
rarely significant, a pattern that suggests that investment and
dependency affect the state's ability to incorporate or effect
changes in the position of women in the labor force. [10]

A third set of intervening mechanisms includes labor-force
composition (bureaucratization), unionization (strikes), distribution of power (power sharing with experts), and the proportion
of the population in urban areas (urbanization). In these
analyses, the level of bureaucratization and strikes have nonsignificant effects. At the same time, power sharing with
experts appears to have a positive effect on women's share of
the labor force. With a reduced number of cases, however,
these results should be treated with caution. This variable
approaches significance in a number of equations and is significant and positive in the TNC investment in extraction equation
(equation 2). An additional effect of this variable is the reduction of the influence of other dependency and investment
indicators. Therefore, the internal power structure is a potential mediating mechanism between investment and dependency
and women's share of economic resources. The socioeconomic
involvement of experts may result in a more equal distribution
of jobs between women and men. [11]

TABLE 4.7

OLS Estimates of the Influence of Investment, Dependency, and Other Intervening Mechanisms on Women's Share of the Labor Force, 1975

Variables	Unstandardized and Standardized Coefficients			
	Women's Share			
MNC INV EX[a]	.02 (.07)	-.05 (-.13)	-.06[b] (.17)	
ΔFOR TRA STR[a]				-29.07[c] (-.21)
GINI[a]	-.34[c] (-.34)			
SUFF EXP[d]				.26[c] (.39)
CENT PLAN ECON				12.18 (.23)
POWER[d]		.64[b] (.35)		
URBPOP[d]			-.16[c] (-.33)	
KWHC[a]	-1.07 (-.16)	.79 (.12)	.86 (.13)	-2.78[c] (-.44)
FEM TERT ED[a]	.08 (.08)	.09 (.09)	.02 (.03)	-.06 (-.07)
ΔTOT LF[d] 60-70	.93 (.21)	.50 (.12)	1.56[c] (.27)	1.33[c] (.25)
Intercept	50.03	16.20	32.65	42.57
R^2	.17	.36	.14	.27
N	67	47	102	86

[a]Measured at t-2, or circa 1965.
[b]$\underline{p}$ < .10.
[c]$\underline{p}$ < .05.
[d]Measured at t-1, or circa 1970.
Note: Variables are defined in Table 4.1. Standardized regression coefficients are in parentheses.

A final variable to consider from this group of intervening mechanisms is urbanization. This variable has a significant and negative effect only in the TNC investment in extraction equation, although coefficients approach significance in the commodity concentration and foreign investment equations. Thus urbanization is indicated as an additional negative influence on women's share of the labor force. This finding provides support for earlier research, which found that women lose access to employment as urbanization increases owing to preferences for male workers in urban areas (Boserup 1970; Youssef 1976; Chaney and Schmink 1980). The effects of urbanization diminish, however, with the inclusion of the centrally planned economies variable.

A fourth set of indicators is organizational and political status of women: variables representing the number of women's groups, experience with suffrage, integration of women in government, and political rights. Only experience with suffrage is consistently significant, and this variable has a positive influence on women's share of the labor force. As is illustrated by equation 4, these effects remain after the inclusion of the centrally planned economies dummy variable. Hence, the longer a nation-state's experience with female suffrage, the greater women's share of the labor force. These effects persist even after controlling for investment/dependency and the level of economic development.

Women's Share of the Industrial and Agricultural Sectors

In most respects, the effects of the four sets of intervening mechanisms on women's share of industry and agriculture are similar to those observed for women's share of the labor force. However, stronger effects for some variables, in particular, income inequality, power sharing, and urbanization, are found (see Table 4.8).

Income inequality has much stronger and negative effects on women's share of the industrial sector than those observed for women's share of the labor force. In the industrial equations, the effects of the foreign trade structure at t-2, foreign investment, and TNC investment in manufacturing are reduced to nonsignificance, while the effects of TNC investment in agriculture remain significant. Here, a unit increase in the Gini results on the average in a -.33 percent decrease in women's share of industry. Thus, most of the negative effects of foreign

TABLE 4.8

OLS Estimates of the Influence of Investment, Dependency, and Other Intervening Mechanisms on Women's Share of Industrial, Agricultural, and Service Sectors, 1975

Variables	Unstandardized and Standardized Coefficients					
	Industrial Share		Agricultural Share		Service Share	
MNC INV AG[a]	-.17[b] (.24)					
FOR DIR INV[a]		.02 (-.09)				
MNC INV MAN[a]				-.02[b] (-.14)		
ΔFOR TRA STR[a]			-19.21[b] (-.19)			
GINI[a]	-.33[b] (-.35)	-.34[b] (-.36)				
POWER[c]			.37[b] (.23)			
URBPOP[c]				-.17[b] (-.24)		
CEN PLAN ECON				7.69[c] (.12)		
% SING WOM[d]						.15[c] (.17)
KWHC[a]	-1.94[b] (-.32)	-1.51 (-.25)	-2.24[b] (-.38)	2.68[b] (.27)	3.13[b] (.35)	2.62[b] (.32)
FEM TERT ED[d]	.25[b] (.29)	.21[c] (.24)	-.08 (-.09)	-.15 (-.11)	.33[b] (.28)	.35[b] (.30)
TOT LF[d]	.35[b] (.35)	.32[b] (.32)	.75[b] (.71)	1.14[b] (.74)	.59[b] (.44)	.56[b] (.46)
Intercept	19.93	21.10	8.72	-49.95	-31.40	-36.80
R^2	.43	.38	.71	.71	.38	.63
N	67	67	45	102	115	72

[a] Measured at t-2, or circa 1965.
[b] $p < .05$.
[c] $p < .10$.
[d] Measured at t-1, or circa 1970.

Note: Variables are defined in Table 4.1. Standardized regression coefficients are in parentheses.

investment on women's share of industry work through the income inequality generated by investment—an additional consequence of dependent development that relies on such investment. At the same time, income inequality has a nonsignificant effect on women's share of agriculture.

Power sharing with experts and urbanization provide additional determinants of women's share of industry and agriculture. Power sharing has a strong positive influence on women's share of industry. The influence of investment and dependency indicators is diminished, with the exception of the variable for change in the trade structure, which becomes significant and negative. In the women's share of agriculture equations, urbanization has a significant negative influence. The investment and dependency indicators remain significant except commodity concentration, which becomes nonsignificant.[12] Although the negative relationship between women's share of agriculture and urbanization is expected, another consideration is other employment opportunities for women. Other research has noted that movement out of agriculture by women in developing countries does not entail movement by women into the modern sector in urban areas (Boserup 1970; Huntington 1975; Chaney and Schmink 1980). Given that industrial jobs are scarce, women frequently can find work only within the informal sector, in unpaid domestic labor or street peddling, for example.

Finally, the role of the state does not have a significant influence on either women's share of industry or agriculture. None of the political status-of-women, bureaucratization, or strike variables is significant. The effects of these variables are subsumed by either the level of development or investment/dependency.

Women's Share of the Service Sector

As noted earlier, investment and dependency indicators have a nonsignificant influence on women's share of the service sector. Likewise, the other specified intervening mechanisms have a nonsignificant influence on this dependent variable. The results of regressing women's share of the service sector on the basic model without the investment/dependency indicators are shown in Table 4.8. Kilowatt hours per capita (KWH/c) has a positive influence on women's service-sector share. This variable is significant, however, only when controlling for the size of the labor force rather than the change in the labor force.

Both labor-force indicators have positive effects on women's share, showing that the size of the labor force and the change in the labor force over time operate to increase women's representation in the service sector. Women's share of tertiary education has a stable positive influence on women's share of service: For each percentage point of change in women's share of education, women's share of the service sector increases by .32 percent. Finally, an alternative determinant of women's service-sector share is the proportion of single women aged fifteen to twenty-four. This variable has a significant and positive effect on women's service-sector share. Thus, the strongest determinants of women's share of the service sector are the size of the labor force, women's education, and KWH/c.

The lack of fit between the specified model and the results for the women's share of service sector equations is puzzling. Two possible explanations are: (1) Women's appearance in the service sector is a function of economic development rather than international economic relationships, or (2) the composition of the service sector is heterogeneous across nation-states. Women's share of the service sector is moderately correlated with other status-of-women variables and the level of economic development. These results suggest that a certain level of economic development needs to be reached before the emergence and growth of the formal service sector takes place. Only then are women drawn extensively into the service sector to meet the demand for increased labor. Further growth in the number of single women spurs this process, as a supply of young and cheap female labor is available to fill positions in the formal service sector. At the same time, variations in definitions of service-sector activity across countries might provide similar results. Two occupations that illustrate the diversity of the service sector are hawking individual cigarettes in a developing country and doing clerical work in a developed country. Only the latter activity, however, is recorded in official statistics, because much of women's service-sector participation in developing countries is hidden in the informal labor market (Tinker 1976). As a result of these factors, economic development is shown to have an effect on women's share of the service sector only after women have entered the formal sector. Investment and dependency, therefore, exhibit negligible effects on women's share of the formal service sector.

DISCUSSION

The pattern of results for the intervening mechanisms indicates that a number of nation-state factors override the effects of investment and dependency on women's economic status. While some direct effects of investment and dependency remain as noted in chapter 2, the intervening mechanisms of income inequality, power sharing, urbanization, and women's political status are also affected by investment and dependency. I suggest that investment and dependency have both direct and indirect effects on the economic status of women. First, classical dependency and foreign investment under dependent development operate directly to reduce women's access to economic resources. Second, these factors operate indirectly through the reduction of the size of the labor force, heightened income inequality, and urbanization, which in turn affect women's share of economic resources.

Direct Effects

These results suggest that classical dependency and dependent development have negative effects on women's share of economic resources. Women's overall share of the labor force and participation rates are affected more by the indicators of classical dependency. Women's shares of the industrial and agricultural sectors, however, are affected by indicators of both classical dependency and dependent development. To illustrate this further, women's share of the labor force is affected by the dependency indicators and by a measure of TNC investment in raw mineral extraction. At the same time, the overall level of foreign investment at an earlier time has a negative effect on women's share, while a flow measure or change in foreign investment has short-term positive effects. In contrast, women's sectoral shares are affected more by indicators of both types of dependency, including TNC investment in manufacturing. Thus, the economic status of women is affected by prior conditions of both classical dependency and dependent development, thereby adding to the consequences of the world economic system noted by other researchers.

As I discussed in chapter 3, the investment data used in these analyses do not distinguish between production for local import substitution and that for export-oriented markets, nor between capital-intensive and labor-intensive investments. What will happen to women's economic status in the long run, given the inflow of export-oriented and labor-intensive facilities by TNCs in the global assembly line, remains to be explored. What these results do indicate is that over time, countries with higher levels of foreign investment and TNC investment in manufacturing have lower proportions of women in the labor force and in the industrial sector. Although very short-term flows in investment enhance women's access to economic resources, in the long run, women's employment may be negatively affected, as is indicated by other research within individual nation-states (Grossman 1978/79; Ehrenreich and Fuentes 1981; Safa 1981). For example, Fernández-Kelly (1983) finds that over time women's economic vulnerability is increased because of the unstable employment of maquiladoras (female assembly line workers). At the same time, additional data on specific forms of TNC investment in the 1970s and 1980s are needed to test more fully the long-term consequences of investment in manufacturing for both women and men.

Additionally, these negative effects of classical dependency and dependent development are found even after controlling for centrally planned economies. Women's overall share of the labor force and participation are directly and negatively affected by changes in the trade structure, earlier levels of commodity concentration, and TNC investment in extraction. If the economic status of women is considered, irrespective of the effects of planned economies, but rather in terms of global patterns of investment, overall foreign investment has a negative effect. Further, if less aggregated measures of women's status are considered, e.g., women's share of the industrial and agricultural sectors, the direct effects of investment and dependency are even stronger—effects that are barely counteracted by centrally planned economies.

Given the pattern of these negative effects from investment and dependency on women's share of both industrial and agricultural sectors, the question arises: To which sectors within the economy are women moving? Evidence from developed nation-states indicates that women are moving into the service sector (Oppenheimer 1970; Blake 1974). Within developing nation-states, however, researchers note that women frequently are unable to find work within the paid service sector, given high levels of male unemployment in the industrial sector and overcrowding within the service sector (Boserup 1970; ICRW 1980b; United Nations 1980). Additional analyses indicate that women's share of the service sector in the peripheral nations falls far below that in the core and semiperipheral nations, 30 percent versus 45 and 37 percent in 1975 (Ward in press). Further, the negative effects of the size of the service sector relative to the total labor force suggest that the extraordinary growth of the service sector, noted by Evans and Timberlake (1980), has had negative effects on women's overall share of the labor force and participation. Thus, if women are either remaining within or moving into the informal sector and if the patterns of investment and dependency continue, women's economic status in developing countries is unlikely to improve.

Indirect Effects

Investment, dependency, and pursuant underdevelopment affect women's share of economic resources indirectly through the size of the labor force, income inequality, urbanization, and other status-of-women variables. Investment and dependency lower the size of the total labor force, net of the level of development.[13] Although the size of the labor force in 1970 and the changes in the size of the labor force raise women's share of economic resources, ultimately these negative effects of investment and dependency on the total labor force suggest that women's employment opportunities could be even more strongly improved if investment and dependency did not lower the size of the labor force relative to the adult population.

As noted by earlier research, heightened income inequality is generated by foreign investment and dependency (Bornschier and Chase-Dunn in press). In this research, income inequality has some inconsistent negative effects on women's overall share of the labor force. In the same equations, the effects of investment are reduced to nonsignificance. These results suggest small but unstable indirect effects of investment through income inequality on women's share of the labor force. Likewise, income inequality has stronger negative effects on women's share of industry, and only the significant direct effects of TNC investment in agriculture remain. Thus, the double negative effects of underdevelopment and investment/dependency on women's share of economic resources are most clearly demonstrated in women's share of industry.

These results support other research from developing nation-states, which notes that, over time, poor women have lost industrial employment. These losses have occurred because of the disruption of traditional industries and women's lack of access to the new industrial employment (Chinchilla 1977; Arizpe 1977; Mazumdar 1979; Chaney and Schmink 1980). Thus, women who already receive a disproportionately small share of income also have limited access to industrial employment. Furthermore, TNC investment in manufacturing often lowers women's share, despite claims by development planners and TNCs. At the same time, one dimension of power equality, power sharing with

experts, may provide one mediating mechanism between investment and income inequality, on the one hand, and women's share
of economic resources, on the other. In a limited number of
cases, higher levels of power sharing with experts elevated
women's share of the labor force and the industrial sector.
Further research is needed to explore these relationships.

The negative effects of urbanization on women's share of
the overall labor force and on women's share of the agricultural
sector are also linked with some of the consequences of investment, dependency, and underdevelopment. One consequence
of investment and dependency is the disproportionate growth
of urban areas within developing nation-states (Kentor 1981;
Timberlake and Kentor 1983). Even with extraordinary levels
of urban growth, the urban employment opportunities for women
are meager. Most women are relegated to the informal sector,
except in Latin America (Boserup 1970; Papanek 1976; Youssef
1976; Chaney and Schmink 1980; Ward in press). Although the
negative effects of urbanization on women's share of agriculture
were expected, it is unclear in what other economic sectors
women in developing countries can find employment, especially
where urbanization has a negative effect on women's overall
employment.

Finally, the other status-of-women variables play a less-
than-important role in the determination of women's share of
labor-force resources. The nonsignificant effects of women's
share of tertiary education on women's share of the labor force
(with the exception of the industrial and service sectors) is
puzzling in light of previous research.

One possible explanation for these negligible effects is
that the tertiary share measure is an inadequate proxy for the
actual educational achievement of women in developing countries
because only a small proportion of the female population is
enrolled in tertiary institutions.[14] Furthermore, the majority
of the illiterate persons in developing countries (two out of
three illiterates on the average) are women: 83 percent of
African and 57 percent of Asian women (Newland 1980). Hence,
a better measure of educational status would be literacy or the
cumulative educational experience of women. Obviously the
lower levels of education and the lack of emphasis on female
education in developing nation-states are major impediments
to women's access to the economic resources generated by
investment and dependency. Other research has found no
direct effects of investment and dependency on women's share
of educational enrollments, with the exception of the negative
effects of TNC investment in extraction (Ward 1982). Women's

educational opportunities may in fact be increased through nation-state incorporation with the world system of trade (Ramirez 1980). The conditions of underdevelopment, however, may impede the financing of educational institutions and the further incorporation of women into these institutions. Consequently, the role of education in facilitating women's access to employment will continue to be negligible until women in developing countries have equal access to education and literacy.

Finally, with the exception of the variable for experience with suffrage, the other status-of-women variables have little influence on women's share of economic resources. The positive influence of suffrage on women's employment indicates that there are long-term effects from earlier adoption of women's suffrage. In contrast, the other political and organizational status-of-women variables are related to the level of development. The effects of women's political and organizational status on women's economic status may be subsumed by their relationship with development and investment/dependency. Further, developing nation-states may adopt equal rights legislation and make efforts to incorporate women within governments in order to appear modern. In reality, these provisions may have only minimal effects on women's access to economic resources. Thus, the negative effects of underdevelopment and investment/dependency on women's share of economic resources are stronger than any positive effects of raising women's political status.

Given the widespread undernumeration of women's economic roles, these reported analyses and results are probably attenuated. Furthermore, owing to the negative influence of investment and dependency on formal labor-force statistics, such results do not bode well for women seeking mobility out of informal labor markets, especially since a hidden effect of investment and dependency is the disruption of women's traditional activities. Thus, within the context of high levels of investment and dependency, women are at a significant economic disadvantage. The next chapter examines the direct effects and implications of this context for fertility.

NOTES

1. The change in the economic status indicators is calculated by comparing the differences between the variables in 1970 and 1975.

2. A measure of state strength is not included in these equations owing to a high relationship between economic develop-

ment and state strength (r = .70). As economic development theoretically is a more important variable, state strength is deleted from the initial equations.

3. Only a few of the increments in R^2 (F) tests were significant, but the results were not readily interpretable because of multicollinearity and large standardized coefficients. (For complete information about the tests see Ward 1982.) Hence, additive results are discussed, but the potential for interaction deserves further research. Only equations with significant investment and dependency variables are reported. A lagged dependent variable is not used in these equations because of the high correlations between the dependent variable measured in 1970 and 1975. (E.g., the correlation between women's share of the labor force in 1970 and 1975 is .99.) This high correlation could indicate that little change in women's share of the labor force and economic sectors and participation occurred. Hence, the effects of the independent variables on the range of variation in the dependent variables in 1975 is examined. Further, for similar reasons, a residual change score for the total labor force variable is used in the overall women's share and participation equations instead of a measure of the total labor force in 1970. Thus, the following results and interpretations are subject to bias by not controlling for the earlier values of the dependent variable. Since theoretically the effects of dependency and investment on women's share of the labor force take place over time, the use of five- to ten-year lags in the independent variables should result in estimates less subject to reciprocal bias than if the dependent and independent variables were measured at the same point in time.

4. These variables are constructed by regressing the level of foreign trade, commodity concentration, or foreign investment at t-1 on the variable at t-2. The time points for the variables used to construct the residual change scores are as follows: foreign trade structure 1965, 1970; commodity concentration, 1965, 1970; foreign investment 1967, 1973.

5. Personal communication, F. Ramirez, March 1982.

6. The effects of the service sector relative to the total labor force remain negative but are reduced to nonsignificance. The changes in commodity concentration and foreign investment variables are not included in these equations owing to missing data for centrally planned economies.

7. The labor-force change score is nonsignificant in these equations. Further, investment and dependency have negative effects on the size of the total labor force (see note 13). Additionally, there is a curvilinear relationship between women's

share of agriculture and level of economic development: The logged development term has a positive but nonsignificant effect on women's share; the squared development term is significant and negative. The other regression results are unchanged, however, with the inclusion of the squared term.

8. Only the results of women's share of the labor force are shown and discussed because the results for women's participation rate are very similar.

9. With the lowered number of cases, multicollinearity is problematic. Thus the centrally planned economies account for only a few of the cases in the regression results. The effects of this dummy variable are reported only when most of the centrally planned economies are in the regression equation.

10. Centrally planned economies are not included in these equations owing to missing data on government revenues as a percentage of the gross domestic product.

11. The centrally planned economies variable is not in these equations owing to the lower number of cases.

12. These significant effects persist even when the squared development variable and the centrally planned economies dummy are in the regression equation.

13. In other analyses, investment and dependency have negative effects on the size of the labor force relative to the total population in 1970, net of the curvilinear influence of development (Ward 1982). A unit change in commodity concentration results in a .12 percent decline in the labor force. Likewise, a unit change in foreign investment and TNC investment in extraction results in a -.04 percent or -.07 percent change. At the same time, a unit change in the foreign trade structure results in a +9.1 percent change in the size of the labor force. Thus, investment and dependency operate indirectly through the size of the labor force.

14. Personal communications, R. Rosenfeld and S. Nuss, March 1982.

5
The Effects of Investment, Dependency, Intervening Mechanisms, and the Status of Women on Fertility

As noted in chapter 2, past research on the determinants of fertility has focused on five factors: modernization or economic development, the world system, income inequality, the educational and economic status of women, and family planning. First, the modernization researchers have assumed that fertility was an individual nation-state problem and that the level of fertility in developing nations compared with developed nations would decline during economic development and the spread of educational institutions and economic resources to the population. At the same time, high infant mortality rates were an intervening factor that operated to raise the level of fertility (Mauldin and Berelson 1978; Tsui and Bogue 1978).

Second, other researchers have argued that the effects of the world economic system have impeded the decline in fertility (Tilly 1978; Repetto 1979; Hout 1980). The effects of trade dependency have operated to keep the value of children high during the processes of underdevelopment (i.e., lowered relative rates of economic growth, heightened income inequality, and disruption of indigenous economies). In turn, economic development does not have a sustained impact in fertility, unless it is accompanied by a decline in trade dependency (Hout 1980). Likewise, foreign or transnational corporation (TNC) investment was predicted to have direct positive effects on fertility and indirect effects through the conditions of underdevelopment. Further, after controlling for dependency, the effects of family planning efforts are diminished or become negligible (Hout 1981).

Third, income inequality, as a consequence of international economic relationships, has been found to lead to higher fertility, net of the influence of economic development (Bhattacharyya 1975; Simon 1977; Repetto 1979). As a result, income inequality has been treated by researchers as an intervening variable between development and fertility.

Fourth, the relationship between the status of women and fertility has received increasing attention (Dixon 1975, 1978b; Kupinsky 1977a; Standing 1978; Youssef 1979, 1982). Although the growth of educational and economic opportunities for women in developed nations has led to a reduction in fertility, these negative relationships might become negligible in developing nations. For example, women in developing countries have lowered access to educational resources. In turn, the education that women do receive frequently does not provide access to employment opportunities in the formal labor force. As a consequence, women have limited access to new ideas and incentives for fertility limitation. The structure of economic opportunities generated by the sexual division of labor for women determines their fertility behavior (Deere, Humphries, and Leon de Leal 1982). If women lack access to formal-sector employment and are relegated to the informal labor markets under the influence of investment and dependency (as noted in chapter 4), women will have little incentive to reduce their fertility. Additionally, children will remain valued economic resources under these conditions (International Center for Research on Women [ICRW] 1980a). The state can play a role in the changing relationships among fertility, the status of women, and the value of children. State provision of social insurance programs may lower the value of children. Legislation also can mandate higher age at marriage and enhance women's legal status and integration in government. Thus, previous research suggests that the state and the organizational and political status of women have a negative influence on fertility (Chaney 1973; Dixon 1975; Hohm 1975; Bruce 1976; Youssef and Hartley 1979).

Fifth, the extension of family planning program efforts has been advocated as a means to lower fertility in developing countries. Researchers have found that family planning programs contribute to the reduction of fertility in developing countries (Mauldin and Berelson 1978; Tsui and Bogue 1978).

Therefore, the effects of family planning and development on fertility should be considered relative to the effects of investment/dependency, the status of women, income inequality, and Coale's (1973) three preconditions for fertility reduction, described in chapter 2. The first precondition is that parents perceive fertility limitation as a conscious and socially acceptable choice. Second, fertility limitation must be socially and economically advantageous. Finally, family planning information and services must be available.

If the effects of investment and dependency are to lower the economic status of women and to perpetuate the high socio-economic value of children, women may not recognize fertility reduction as a conscious choice or perceive it as socially and economically advantageous. Further, if investment and dependency result in heightened income inequality, this variable becomes another intervening factor between development and fertility. Thus, the conditions under investment/dependency and the lowered status of women may impede efforts to bring about continued reduction of fertility through socioeconomic pressures toward high fertility. These factors have not been incorporated in previous analyses.

The basic model for the determination of fertility should include indicators of investment or dependency that are predicted to have a positive effect on fertility, an indicator of the level of economic development that should have a negative effect on fertility, and, finally, indicators of the educational and economic status of women that for the most part should have negative effects on fertility (see Figures 2.2 and 3.2). In this research several indicators of the economic status of women are used: women's share of the labor force and economic sectors and women's participation rate. (See chapter 4 for the determinants of women's economic status.) In general, the overall indicators, women's share of the total labor force and the participation rate, are expected to have weaker negative effects on fertility behavior than the measures of women's share of the industrial and service sectors, while women's share of the agricultural sector should have positive effects on fertility.

Three major intervening variables are indicated from the literature review: infant mortality, income inequality, and family planning. Additional or alternative intervening variables are the strength of the state, existence of social insurance programs, the proportion of single women aged fifteen to twenty-four, and indicators of women's organizational and political status. Within the basic model, infant mortality and income inequality are expected to have positive effects on fertility, while family planning is expected to have negative effects. Further, the intervening variables for the state and the status of women are expected to have negative effects on fertility.

To examine the influence of these specified variables on fertility behavior, past patterns of fertility and correlations between the independent variables and the fertility dependent variable are discussed. Then a three-part research strategy

is used. Hout (1980) proposes that dependency and development interact in their influence on fertility and that development
has a curvilinear effect on fertility; this possibility is examined
as a first analytical step. If no interaction or curvilinear effects
are found, then, second, the additive effects of the variables
in the basic model are estimated, using multiple regression
analysis. Third, the relative effects of the major intervening
variables are estimated through their inclusion in the basic
model, followed by the estimation of the effects of the alternative
intervening variables.

DATA AND CORRELATIONS

From 1968 to 1975, for a group of 126 nation-states, the
level of fertility behavior as measured by the total fertility rate
declined from 5,069 to 4,620 births per 1,000 women over their
lifetime. (See Table 5.1 for sample means, standard deviations,
and correlations.)
The patterns of fertility behavior found in developed and
developing nations are predicted to be related to investment/
dependency, the status of women, and intervening variables.
In general, the relationships between fertility in 1975 and the
independent variables are as predicted (see Table 5.1). Of
the investment, dependency, and development indicators,
commodity concentration is positively correlated with fertility
($r = .55$), and the other indicators of investment have smaller
positive relationships, with the exception of the change in
foreign investment, which has a negative relationship with
fertility ($r = -.46$). In contrast, the general level of economic
development or energy usage has a strong negative relationship
with fertility ($r = -.78$), followed by the negative relationship
of foreign trade structure ($r = -.63$). Thus, while economic
development is related to lower fertility, investment and dependency provide pressures that may counteract such negative
relationships.

Status-of-Women Variables

The negative relationships between fertility and the status-
of-women variables are somewhat smaller than those exhibited
by development and investment variables. Women's share of
education at the secondary and tertiary levels has negative
correlations with fertility ($r = -.68$ and $-.61$). At the same

TABLE 5.1

Number of Cases, Means, Standard Deviations, and Correlations

Varia-bles	TFR	LTFR	KWHC	TRSTR	CMCON	FDI	MNCAG	MNCEX	MNCM	GINI	ΔTRS	ΔCOM	ΔFDI	DCPE	GGR	PWLF	WLFP
N	126	126	126	104	87	114	114	114	114	75	104	79	105	126	113	126	126
X̄	4620.17	5069.36	5.79	-.38	43.23	54.97	7.55	20.00	16.40	44.71	-1.32E-16	5.59E-15	3.10E-14	.06	21.77	29.81	40.52
Sd.	1809.67	1739.10	1.76	.33	22.95	43.28	16.03	35.22	15.50	10.26	.08	9.29	26.97	.24	9.19	12.28	21.71
TFR	1.00																
LTFR	.956	1.00															
KWHC	-.780	-.759	1.00														
TRSTR	-.633	-.681	.498	1.00													
CMCON	-.533	-.575	-.463	-.641	1.00												
FDI	.198	.214	-.012	-.382	-.324	1.00											
MNCAG	.203	.202	-.185	-.276	.221	.506	1.00										
MNCEX	.285	.300	-.064	-.370	.548	.753	.316	1.00									
MNCM	-.150	-.133	.172	-.114	-.121	.604	.324	.157	1.00								
GINI	.621	.662	-.401	-.499	.425	.436	.255	.432	.157	1.00							
ΔTRS	-.005	-.020	.052	-.000	-.173	-.138	-.088	-.134	-.016	.118	1.00						
ΔCOM	.120	.137	-.019	-.038	.000	.140	-.079	.248	-.137	.106	-.124	1.00					
ΔFDI	-.458	-.436	.308	.375	-.367	-.000	-.165	-.154	-.228	-.270	.014	-.079	1.00				
DCPE	-.298	-.361	.295	.280	-.214	-.350	-.130	-.188	-.292	-.555	-.163	.010	-.030	1.00			
GGR	-.595	-.599	.702	.398	.261	.084	-.205	.010	-.125	-.405	-.048	.162	.221	.054	1.00		
LPWLF	-.245	-.296	-.034	-.204	-.270	-.221	.037	-.242	.044	-.275	-.212	-.031	.209	.298	-.062	1.00	
LWLFP	-.113	-.165	-.161	.139	-.188	-.205	.074	-.221	.016	-.230	-.216	-.040	.156	.266	-.136	.972	1.00
LPWAG	-.077	-.146	-.185	.187	-.195	-.303	.029	-.224	-.154	-.231	-.146	.102	.070	.316	-.169	.841	.843
LPWSER	-.415	-.424	.388	.195	-.294	-.031	-.026	-.109	.101	-.189	-.100	-.068	.265	.245	.173	.467	.355
LPWIND	-.159	-.186	.012	.236	-.129	-.322	-.162	-.248	-.101	-.335	-.100	-.277	.155	.247	.173	.533	.515
SOCINS	-.787	-.794	.776	.552	-.498	-.107	-.245	-.293	-.218	-.495	-.017	-.106	.333	.290	-.144	.082	-.011
PF3ED	-.614	-.595	.613	.297	-.274	-.171	-.061	-.176	.241	-.469	.010	-.214	.166	.324	-.653	.000	-.106
WGPS	-.341	-.292	.391	.419	-.314	-.187	-.205	-.183	-.066	-.047	-.045	.066	.123	-.127	.302	.053	-.022
SUFFEX	-.655	-.656	.613	.298	-.360	-.194	-.161	-.323	.180	.471	-.077	-.139	.287	.177	.316	.184	.097
WGVINT	-.399	-.391	.508	.360	-.301	-.115	-.058	-.204	.079	-.300	.101	-.124	.287	-.149	.549	-.004	-.056
POLINX	-.115	-.181	.154	-.233	-.047	-.295	-.027	-.213	-.204	-.247	-.163	-.124	.236	-.261	.345	-.004	.004
IMR	.827	.786	-.818	-.506	.533	.102	.105	.290	-.213	.550	-.163	-.213	.055	-.455	.028	-.006	.004
FAMPLAN	-.765	-.585	.488	-.179	-.214	-.084	-.214	-.046	.012	-.267	-.033	-.007	.254	.000	-.522	-.068	.109
PSW1524	-.642	-.624	.539	.466	-.500	.113	-.155	-.245	-.295	-.295	.010	-.029	.425	.058	.375	.109	.013

(continued)

Table 5.1 (continued)

Varia-bles	LPWAG	LPWSER	LPWIND	SOCINS	LPF3ED	WGPS	SUFFEX	WGVINT	POLINX	IMR	FAMPLAN	PSW1524
N	126	126	126	109	115	95	109	78	126	114	66	74
X̄	26.41	33.10	20.16	80.94	27.96	3.99	23.43	5.94	1.25	92.42	6.42	2.41
Sd.	17.35	15.83	12.69	47.52	12.62	3.07	15.97	2.73	1.15	59.41	7.93	14.93
TFR												
LTFR												
KWHC												
TRSTR												
CMCON												
FDI												
MNCAG												
MNCEX												
MNCM												
GINI												
ΔTRS												
ΔCOM												
ΔFDI												
DCPE												
GGR												
LPWLF												
LWLFP												
LPWAG	1.00											
LPWSER	.077	1.00										
LPWIND	.320	.479	1.00									
SOCINS	-.094	.362	.089	1.00								
LPF3ED	-.154	.396	.141	.556	1.00							
WGPS	-.096	.246	.044	.228	.254	1.00						
SUFFEX	-.023	.394	.139	.636	.485	.317	1.00					
WGVINT	-.185	.293	.126	.457	.500	.369	.418	1.00				
POLINX	.034	.063	.181	.271	.222	-.023	.007	.270	1.00			
IMR	.145	-.405	-.049	-.700	-.634	-.289	.613	-.474	-.124	1.00		
FAMPLAN	-.147	.147	.144	.213	-.465	-.348	.370	-.404	-.081	-.629	1.00	
PSW1524	.076	.489	.322	.558	.489	.104	.380	.251	-.013	-.744	.412	1.00

Variable definitions (terms in parentheses are variable names used in regression tables)

TFR	total fertility rate, 1975
LTFR	lagged total fertility rate, 1968
KWHC	logged kilowatt hours per capita, 1965 (KWHC)
TRSTR	foreign trade structure (FOR TRA STR)
CMCON	commodity concentration, 1965 (COM CONC)
FDI	foreign direct investment, 1967 (FOR DIR INV)
MNCAG	multinational (MNC) investment in agriculture, 1967
MNCEX	MNC investment in extraction, 1967 (MNC INV EXT)
MNCM	MNC investment in manufacturing, 1967
GINI	income inequality, 1967 (GINI)
ΔTRS	residual change score foreign trade structure, 1965-1970
ΔCOM	residual change score commodity concentration, 1965-1970
ΔFDI	residual change score foreign direct investment, 1967-1973 (FOR DIR INV)
DCPE	centrally planned economies
GGR	government revenues as a percentage of the gross domestic product, 1970
LPWLF	women's share of the labor force, 1970 (FEM SHA LF)
LWLFP	women's labor-force participation rate, 1970 (FEM LFP)
LPWAG	women's share of the agricultural sector, 1970 (FEM SHA AG)
LPWSER	women's share of the service sector, 1970 (FEM SHA SERV)
LPWIND	women's share of the industrial sector, 1970 (FEM SHA IND)
SOCINS	social insurance program experience, 1970 (SOC INS PROG)
LPF3ED	women's share of tertiary education, 1970 (FEM TERT ED)
WGPS	number of women's groups, 1970
SUFFEX	years experience with suffrage, 1970
WGVINT	integration of women in government, 1970
POLINX	political rights index, 1970
IMR	infant mortality rate, 1968 (INF MORT)
FAMPLAN	family planning program effort, 1972 (FAM PLAN)
PSW1524	proportion of single women aged 15-24, 1970 (%SING WOM)

time, women's shares of the labor force and service sector
have the highest correlations with fertility among the major
economic status indicators ($r = -.25$ and $-.42$). Last, certain
organizational and political status-of-women variables have
negative correlations with fertility: the number of women's
groups ($r = -.34$), experience with suffrage ($r = -.66$), the
integration of women in government ($r = -.40$), and women's
political rights index ($r = -.12$). The correlations of the organizational and political variables with fertility are significant,
with the exception of the political rights correlation.

Intervening Mechanisms

Certain intervening variables are also of interest in the
process of fertility determination. The level of income inequality
is positively related to fertility, and the level of infant mortality
has an even stronger relationship ($r = .62$ and $.83$). The
strength of the state is directly and negatively correlated with
fertility ($r = -.59$); the provision of social insurance program
experience has a similar negative relationship ($r = -.78$).
The proportion of single women aged fifteen to twenty-four
is negatively correlated with fertility ($r = -.64$). Additionally,
family planning program effort is strongly and negatively
related to fertility ($r = -.76$).

Therefore, an examination of the zero-order relationships
between fertility and the specified variables indicates a moderate
congruence between the theoretical relationships proposed in
chapter 2 and the empirical indicators. I evaluate the relative
influence of the independent variables on fertility behavior in
the next few sections by first examining the influence of
investment/dependency and status of women on fertility and
then examining the relative influence of these factors while
controlling for intervening mechanisms.

REGRESSION ANALYSIS

The Influence of Investment/Dependency
and the Status of Women

The basic model for testing the influence of investment/
dependency and the status of women on fertility consists of
regressing the total fertility rate in 1975 on an indicator of
investment/dependency, women's share of tertiary education

and economic resources, and energy usage. (Countries used
in analysis are shown in Appendix B.) Then the effects of
other intervening variables are examined by entering these
variables into the basic regression model. As a first step in
analysis, I examined the possibility of interaction and curvilinear
relationships among investment/dependency, development, and
fertility, net of the influence of the status of women, in light
of the research by Hout (1980). No significant interaction
between investment/dependency and development or a curvilinear relationship between development and fertility was found.[1]
Thus, in the remaining analyses, additive effects are reported.

The results of the basic model, that is, of regressing
fertility on separate investment/dependency indicators, women's
share of the labor force or women's participation rate, women's
share of tertiary education, and energy usage (development),
are found in Tables 5.2 and 5.3 ("a" columns).[2] Overall,
commodity concentration, foreign investment, and TNC investment in extraction have positive direct effects on fertility.
Greater diversity of the foreign trade structure and change in
foreign investment lower fertility, as shown in Tables 5.2 and
5.3. Concurrently, the level of development has the strongest
negative influence, along with the smaller negative effects of
women's share of tertiary education and women's share of the
labor force and participation rate. For example, a one percent
change in women's share of the labor force results in a 29 to
49 birth decline per 1,000 women (Table 5.2). Women's share
of the labor force has negative, albeit smaller, significant effects
on fertility (see the unstandardized coefficients). The difference in the size of the effects of the two economic status variables
on fertility indicates that women's share of resources is more
important than women's participation rate.

Other indicators of women's economic status include women's
share of the agricultural, industrial, and service sectors. The
sector indicators represent less aggregated measures of women's
economic status. In contrast to earlier predictions, the sectoral
status-of-women indicators all have smaller but similar negative
effects compared to women's share of the labor force on fertility.
In an analysis not reported here, the predicted hierarchy of
effects from the women's share of economic sectors was found
to be unsupported. A comparison of the unstandardized coefficients reveals that women's share of agriculture has the
next strongest negative effects after women's share of the total
labor force, followed by the effects of women's share of industry
and the service sector. These coefficients range in size from
-.12 to -.28 percent (Ward 1982). As to the hierarchy of sector

TABLE 5.2

Ordinary Least Squares (OLS) Estimates of the Influence of Investment/Dependency, Women's Share of the Labor Force, and Infant Mortality on Fertility, 1975

Variables	Unstandardized and Standardized Coefficients									
	a	b	a	b	a	b	a	b	a	b
FOR TRA STR†	-1173.83** (-.22)	-905.17** (-.17)								
COM CONC†			14.52* (.18)	8.91* (.11)						
FOR DIR INV†					3.47* (.08)	2.18 (.05)				
MNC INV EXT†							8.61** (.16)	4.68* (.08)		
ΔFOR DIR INV‡									-9.87** (-.15)	-6.30* (-.10)
INF MORT‡		13.62** (.43)		10.44** (.32)		10.91** (.35)		9.48** (.30)		9.24** (.30)
KWHC†	-656.29** (-.63)	-374.82** (-.35)	-720.64** (-.65)	-526.38** (-.47)	-772.88** (-.73)	-531.44** (-.50)	-773.99** (-.73)	-536.84** (-.53)	-723.50** (-.69)	-545.66** (-.52)
FEM TERT ED‡	-26.78** (-.18)	-15.03* (-.10)	-28.07** (-.18)	-15.00 (-.09)	-22.54** (-.15)	-11.75 (-.08)	-20.92** (-.14)	-12.02 (-.08)	-29.33** (-.20)	-18.03** (-.12)
FEM SHA LF‡	-28.73** (-.18)	-29.31** (-.19)	-42.05** (-.27)	-40.71 (-.27)	-45.29** (-.30)	-42.47** (-.29)	-42.17** (-.28)	-41.56** (-.28)	-46.97** (-.31)	-44.60** (-.30)
Intercept	9495.48	6446.35	10258.17	8001.75	10977.79	8213.61	10816.23	8525.77	11077.42	8777.25
R^2	.79	.85	.81	.84	.79	.85	.81	.85	.79	.84
N	95	90	82	78	105	99	105	99	97	92

†Measured circa 1965.
‡Measured circa 1970.
*p < .10.
**p < .05.
Note: Variables are defined in Table 5.1. Standardized regression coefficients are in parentheses. "a" columns depict basic model; "b" columns include infant mortality.

TABLE 5.3

OLS Estimates of the Influence of Investment/Dependency, Women's Labor-Force Participation, and Infant Mortality on Fertility, 1975

Variables	Unstandardized and Standardized Coefficients									
	a	b	a	b	a	b	a	b	a	b
FOR TRA STR†	-1196.32** (-.22)	-930.55** (-.17)								
COM CONC†			15.67** (.19)	10.31** (.12)						
FOR DIR INV†					3.52* (.08)	2.20 (.05)				
MNC INV EXT†							8.66** (.16)	4.54* (.08)		
ΔFOR DIR INV†									-10.50** (-.16)	-6.98** (-.11)
INF MORT‡		13.49** (.42)		10.27** (.31)		11.19** (.35)		9.81** (.31)		9.31** (.30)
KWHC†	-668.66** (-.64)	-338.52** (-.37)	-735.37** (-.66)	-541.53** (-.49)	-799.79** (-.76)	-549.44** (-.52)	-798.39** (-.76)	-579.59** (-.55)	-749.33** (-.71)	-566.64** (-.54)
FEM TERT ED‡	-28.38** (-.19)	-16.96** (-.11)	-30.72** (-.19)	-17.60* (-.11)	-24.92** (-.17)	-13.79* (-.09)	-22.55** (-.15)	-14.06* (-.09)	-32.16** (-.22)	-20.61** (-.14)
FEM LFP‡	-14.41** (-.16)	-14.66** (-.17)	-22.80** (-.25)	-21.70 (-.24)	-24.27** (-.28)	-22.69** (-.27)	-22.32** (-.26)	-22.10** (-.26)	-25.72** (-.30)	-24.15** (-.29)
Intercept	9315.49	6292.59	10038.93	7786.96	10833.07	8003.76	10668.17	8304.76	10948.3	8615.3
R²	.78	.84	.80	.83	.78	.84	.80	.83	.78	.83
N	95	90	82	79	105	99	105	99	97	92

†Measured circa 1965.
‡Measured circa 1970.
*p < .10.
**p < .05.

Note: Variables are defined in Table 5.1. Standardized regression coefficients are in parentheses. "a" columns depict basic model; "b" columns include infant mortality.

effects, these results suggest that if women have a greater
share of the agriculture sector, they will reduce their fertility
over and above the effects of women's share of industry. The
smaller effects of women's share of the service sector are explained, in part, by the correlation between development and
women's share of the service sector (r = .39); in other words,
some of the service-sector effects on fertility are shared by
the effects of development.[3] Because of the stronger effects
of the variable for female share of the labor force on fertility,
however, this variable is used in the remainder of the analyses
as an indicator of women's economic status. Where the results
differ for the equations containing the other economic status-of-
women variables, these differences are noted.

Thus, from these analyses using the basic model, the level
of economic development has the strongest negative effects on
fertility. At the same time, status-of-women and investment/
dependency indicators have smaller but independent effects on
fertility, net of the level of development. The economic status
of women has a relatively stronger negative effect than women's
share of tertiary education. This latter relationship could result
in part from the high correlation between development and
women's share of education. Some investment/dependency
indicators work to raise fertility, while others, such as the
diversity of foreign trade structure and the change in the level
of foreign investment, have negative effects that are either strong
or weak on fertility. To this we can add the negative influence
of investment/dependency on the economic status of women,
which in turn affects the relationship between the status of
women and fertility by lowering women's share of the labor force
and economic sectors. The importance of these findings, however, is that although the effects of investment/dependency
and the status of women are small, these factors have significant
effects, net of development. In other words, the level of development incompletely represents the effects of these factors on
fertility. Hence, it is an unsuitable proxy for the effects of
status of women, investment, and dependency on fertility.
Thus, analyses that omit these variables are subject to specification error. These regression results, however, need to be
evaluated relative to the effects of the major intervening variables, i.e., infant mortality, income inequality, and family planning
programs.

Intervening Mechanisms

In this section, I evaluate the effects of the major intervening variables by entering each intervening variable separately

into the equations and then by comparing their effects, net of the other intervening variables.[4] Then I examine the influence of alternative intervening variables: the state, social insurance programs, the proportion of single women, and other political and organizational status of women variables.

Infant Mortality

When the infant mortality rate is included in the basic equations (see "b" columns in Tables 5.2 and 5.3), this variable has a strong positive effect on fertility, and the direct effects of investment and dependency variables are reduced (see, for example, Table 5.2). The effects of commodity concentration and TNC investment in extraction are small but significant. Foreign trade structure and change in foreign investment maintain their negative influence, and foreign investment becomes nonsignificant. The relative influence of development declines, but it remains the strongest determinant of fertility followed by the effects of infant mortality. Women's share of the labor force is consistently significant and negative in these equations. Women's share of tertiary education becomes nonsignificant.[5]

Therefore, when infant mortality is introduced into the basic model, the effects of investment and dependency are reduced, suggesting potential indirect effects of these variables through infant mortality on fertility behavior. For example, commodity concentration has a positive correlation with infant mortality ($r = .53$), which suggests a potential relationship between dependency and social settings.[6] The other investment and dependency effects are reduced in size, which might indicate that infant mortality is an intervening factor that surpasses the direct influence of investment/dependency on fertility. The strength of infant mortality as an intervening variable is further demonstrated by the reduction of the development effects on fertility.

A partial explanation for the reduction of the status-of-women effects is the multicollinearity between education and infant mortality ($r = -.64$). Further, the level of infant mortality diminishes the potential negative influence of women's economic status on fertility. Consequently, if a high level of infant mortality prevails, the economic status of women is less able to counteract the strong pressures toward high fertility provided by the infant mortality rate. Thus, when the effects of investment/dependency and infant mortality are controlled, previous negative relationships between the economic status of women and fertility are reduced, with women's share of the labor force having the largest net effects in comparison with the other economic status-of-women indicators.

Income Inequality

Another major intervening variable is one of the consequences of investment and dependency: income inequality.
The effects of income inequality on fertility relative to the other
previously specified independent variables (with the exception
of infant mortality) are shown in Table 5.4 ("a" columns).
For example, in the equations that include women's share of
the labor force as a measure of women's economic status, the
positive and significant effects from a unit change in income
inequality range from 29 to 50 additional births per 1,000 women.
At the same time, the strong negative effects of development
are only slightly reduced across all equations. The effects of
foreign investment and TNC investment in extraction are reduced
to nonsignificance, and the small positive effects of change in
foreign investment disappear. In contrast, the direct effects
of dependency measures remain significant where an increase
in the diversity of foreign trade structure leads to a decline in
fertility; an increase in commodity concentration leads to an
increase in fertility. Thus, the effects of investment on fertility
become nonsignificant when controlling for income inequality,
while the effects of classical dependency indicators remain
significant. Further, the effects of women's share of the labor
force become nonsignificant in the commodity concentration
equation; women's share of education has consistently small
and negative effects on fertility.

Income inequality, therefore, has small positive effects on
fertility; the effects of other independent variables are reduced,
in particular, the influence of all indicators of women's economic
status.[7] This latter effect of income inequality suggests that
countries experiencing high levels of income inequality and
investment/dependency may find that previous negative relationships between the economic status of women and fertility are
reduced or become negligible, especially in regard to the effects
of women's participation and share of economic sectors. For
example, income inequality, which in chapter 4 was found to
reduce women's share of industry, also reduces the effects of
this variable on fertility. As a result, education has a greater
influence on fertility than on women's economic status. The
reduced investment and dependency effects could be the result
of the causal relationship demonstrated in past research, where
higher levels of investment/dependency have led to heightened
income inequality (Chase-Dunn 1975; Bornschier, Chase-Dunn,
and Rubinson 1978). Finally, the strong effects of development
on fertility net of income inequality are in contradiction to the
findings of Repetto (1979), who argued that income inequality
has an equally strong influence on fertility. Thus, the small

TABLE 5.4

OLS Estimates of the Influence of Investment/Dependency, Status of Women, Income Inequality, and Family Planning Programs on Fertility, 1975

Variables	Unstandardized and Standardized Coefficients									
	a	b	a	b	a	b	a	b	a	b
FOR TRA STR†	-963.52** (-.20)	-332.83 (-.06)								
COM CONC†			13.55 (.16)	61.34 (.01)						
FOR DIR INV†					.71 (.02)	-.78 (-.03)				
MNC INV EXT†							5.00 (.09)	.89 (.03)		
ΔFOR DIR INV‡									-5.06 (.08)	-.87 (-.02)
GINI†		29.90** (.15)		50.48** (.25)		51.09** (.28)		43.29** (.24)		72.51** (.34)
FAM PLAN‡	-82.41** (-.53)		-72.83** (-.48)		-78.31** (-.52)		-76.50** (-.51)		-76.77** (-.51)	
KWHC†	-663.66** (-.59)	-345.78** (-.35)	-629.81** (-.59)	-271.72** (-.32)	-736.17** (-.62)	-285.92** (-.33)	-744.80* (-.63)	-321.18** (-.37)	-714.67** (-.59)	-301.96** (-.35)
FEM TERT ED‡	-27.21** (-.17)	-17.35* (-.16)	-23.76** (-.14)	-24.11** (-.27)	-21.90** (-.13)	-20.17** (-.22)	-23.17** (-.14)	-19.20** (-.21)	-27.19** (-.16)	-19.65** (-.21)
FEM SHA LF‡	-16.93** (-.09)	-23.58** (-.24)	-15.34 (-.09)	-23.41** (-.29)	-20.07* (-.11)	-29.94** (-.35)	-21.15** (-.12)	-30.97** (-.37)	-27.50** (-.15)	-30.08** (-.36)
Intercept	7933.57	8645.56	6919.90	8705.06	7805.00	8896.81	8212.96	8990.73	7029.08	8905.69
R^2	.84	.71	.85	.66	.83	.71	.83	.71	.86	.71
N	61	66	56	57	67	72	67	72	62	72

†Measured circa 1965.
‡Measured circa 1970.
*$p < .10$.
**$p < .05$.

Note: Variables are defined in Table 5.1. Standardized regression coefficients are in parentheses. "a" columns include family planning; "b" columns include GINI.

direct effects of commodity concentration and income inequality only slightly impede the reduction of fertility; other previously negative relationships between the status of women and fertility are lowered.

Family Planning Program Effort

The effects of family planning program effort while controlling for the other independent variables in the basic model (except infant mortality and income inequality) are shown in Table 5.4 ("b" columns). Since this variable is available only for developing nations, these results should be viewed with caution due to the truncated range of countries.[8] Family planning program effort has a strong negative influence on fertility. A unit change in program effort lowers the number of births ranging from 72 to 82 births per 1,000 women. The effects of development are reduced but remain the next strongest determinant of fertility after family planning, while the effects of investment/dependency on fertility become nonsignificant. The status-of-women variables remain significant, including the effects of women's share of tertiary education, although this latter variable becomes less important than women's share of the labor force in the determination of fertility.

Hernandez (1981), however, notes that the effectiveness of this family planning variable is overstated unless other social and development variables that may enhance the effectiveness of family planning programs are controlled in regression analyses. Likewise, I argue that intervening variables such as infant mortality and income inequality need to be controlled in order to assess the relative effectiveness of family planning. The effects of program effort are assessed relative to the level of income inequality and infant mortality in Table 5.5 ("a" and "b" columns). Additionally, the relative influence of income inequality net of the effects of infant mortality is examined ("c" columns).[9]

Family Planning Versus Income Inequality. When the family planning variable is included in the same basic equation with income inequality, both variables are significant, with effects in the predicted direction (see Table 5.5, "a" columns). The nonsignificant effects of investment and dependency variables remain as in the previous equations in Table 5.4; women's share of the labor force is negative but nonsignificant in the commodity concentration equations. In each equation, the standardized regression coefficients indicate that family planning program effort has a stronger influence on fertility than income

inequality, but there is a reduction in the size of the family
planning unstandardized coefficients from the coefficients observed in Table 5.4. Meanwhile, the effects of economic development remain strong and negative. The negative effects of
women's share of tertiary education are consistently significant
and small.

Family Planning Versus Infant Mortality. When the family
planning variable is included in the equations with the infant
mortality variable, the infant mortality variable becomes nonsignificant, albeit negative with the exception of the trade
structure equation (see Table 5.5, "b" columns). The combined
influence of family planning and infant mortality substantially
reduces the influence of development on fertility. The nonsignificant effects of investment and dependency variables
persist. The status-of-women variables are significant, although
women's share of the labor force is a stronger determinant of
fertility than is education in these equations. Thus, in this
limited group of countries, the positive effects of infant mortality
on fertility and the negative effects of development are reduced
if family planning program effort is taken into consideration.
In other words, family planning programs can overcome the
positive effects of infant mortality on fertility; these programs
can also surpass the effects of development on fertility.

Income Inequality Versus Infant Mortality. Finally, with the
inclusion of both income inequality and infant mortality in the
same equations (see Table 5.5, "c" columns), both variables
are significant and have positive effects on fertility, with the
exception of the trade structure equation, where income inequality is nonsignificant. The standardized regression coefficients
indicate that infant mortality has a stronger effect than income
inequality on fertility. As in Table 5.4, investment and dependency have nonsignificant effects on fertility, while the
influence of women's share of the labor force is reduced and
becomes nonsignificant in the trade structure equation. Development and education remain significant and negative for all
equations except the commodity concentration equation, where
education becomes nonsignificant.

From the findings in Tables 5.4 and 5.5, family planning
program effort is important in the reduction of fertility, net
of the effects of income inequality, infant mortality, and
investment/dependency. These effects of family planning,
however, are lowered if social and economic factors such as
income inequality are included in the analyses (as can be seen
by comparing the family planning standardized coefficients

TABLE 5.5

OLS Estimates of the Influence of Investment/Dependency, Women's Share of the Labor Force, Gini, Family Planning Program Efforts, and Infant Mortality on Fertility, 1975

Variables	Unstandardized and Standardized Coefficients								
	a	b	c	a	b	c	a	b	c
FOR TRA STR†	-444.63 (-.08)	-254.41 (-.05)	-709.01* (-.14)						
COM CONC†				3.56 (.07)	-1.58 (-.03)	8.84 (.10)			
FOR DIR INV†							-.62 (-.02)	-1.46 (-.06)	.10 (-.10)
MNC INV EXT†									
ΔFOR DIR INV‡									
KWHC†	-532.51** (-.50)	-189.92* (-.19)	-426.16** (-.38)	-461.70** (-.45)	-168.72* (-.20)	-438.86* (-.37)	-475.52* (-.45)	-186.32* (-.21)	-467.95** (-.40)
GINI†	37.39** (.22)		19.78 (.10)	37.45* (.25)		33.50** (.16)	37.05** (.22)		29.57** (.16)
FAM PLAN‡	-45.97** (-.29)	-81.48** (-.54)		-55.10** (-.36)	-77.18** (-.55)		-64.46** (-.40)	-77.93** (-.54)	
INF MORT‡		5.89** (.23)	12.65** (.37)		2.88 (.12)	13.34** (.38)		3.15 (.14)	14.04** (.40)
FEM TERT ED‡	-27.44** (-.27)	-10.48 (-.10)	-17.70* (-.11)	-24.83** (-.27)	-16.65* (-.20)	-8.62 (-.05)	-25.35** (-.24)	-14.96** (-.17)	-9.39 (-.06)
FEM SHA LF‡	-18.69* (-.16)	-23.12** (-.24)	-11.64 (-.06)	-17.72 (-.19)	-20.71** (-.28)	-16.52** (-.10)	-22.00** (-.20)	-27.15** (-.34)	-21.88** (-.12)
Intercept	7673.32	7096.40	5570.87	7416.43	7615.18	4802.43	7907.37	7885.38	5677.13
R^2	.77	.76	.90	.69	.68	.89	.77	.74	.88
N	39	63	57	35	55	53	41	70	63

	a	b	c	a	b	c
FOR TRA STR†	1.09 (.03)	-1.57 (-.05)	.30 (-.01)			-1.45 (-.02)
COM CONC†						
FOR DIR INV†						
MNC INV EXT†				2.22 (.05)		
ΔFOR DIR INV‡					-.50 (-.01)	
KWHC†	-508.08** (-.48)	-180.74** (.03)	-470.15** (-.40)	-488.80** (-.46)	-219.76** (-.25)	-543.78** (-.46)
GINI†	35.72** (.21)		29.38** (.16)	36.66** (.21)		50.72** (.22)
FAM PLAN‡		-77.74** (-.54)			-76.25** (-.53)	
INF MORT‡	-63.44** (-.39)	3.48 (.15)	13.94** (.39)	-66.26** (-.41)	3.01 (.13)	10.16** (.29)
FEM TERT ED‡	-25.32** (-.24)	-14.77** (-.16)	-9.52 (-.06)	-25.12** (-.24)	-14.28* (-.16)	-15.35 (-.09)
FEM SHA LF‡	-23.98** (-.22)	-27.56** (-.34)	-21.95** (-.12)	-23.78** (-.22)	-28.07** (-.35)	-27.34* (-.15)
Intercept	8124.22	7783.63	5712.59	8025.11	7975.24	5784.97
R²	.77	.74	.88	.77	.73	.88
N	41	70	63	41	70	58

†Measured circa 1965.
‡Measured circa 1970.
*p < .10.
**p < .05.
Note: Variables are defined in Table 5.1. "a" columns include Gini and family planning; "b" columns include family planning and infant mortality; "c" columns include Gini and infant mortality.

between Tables 5.4 and 5.5). Further, the combined effects
of infant mortality and income inequality on fertility in a more
economically diverse group of countries indicate that these two
factors provide underlying pressures toward high fertility.
Thus, net of investment and dependency, the strongest predict-
ors of fertility are development, family planning, infant mortality,
and income inequality, even though the effects of development
on fertility are reduced after controlling for family planning
and infant mortality.

Other Intervening Mechanisms

The role of the state, provision of social insurance programs, and other indicators of the status of women are mentioned
as negative determinants of fertility behavior. In regression
results not reported here, when a measure of state strength
(e.g., government revenues as a percent of the gross domestic
product) is included in the basic regression model with infant
mortality, the state has a negative and significant influence on
fertility. However, if either income inequality or family planning
effort is included in the equations, the state effects become
nonsignificant. These latter results can be attributed, first,
to the measures of state family planning involvement in the family
planning variable, and, second, to the fact that the effects of
income inequality suppress the negative effects of state strength
on fertility (Ward 1982).
A state, however, can affect fertility rates through the
provision of social insurance programs that, in effect, lower
the value of children through old-age security programs (Friedlander and Silver 1967; Hohm 1975). Social insurance program
experience has a negative influence on fertility, even after
controlling for the separate effects of infant mortality and
income inequality in the basic regression equation; but social
insurance experience has a nonsignificant effect when family
planning effort is controlled for (Ward 1982). Hence, nation-
states with a history of social insurance programs have lower
rates of fertility, net of the effects of development and other
specified variables. These effects disappear in the limited
sample of developing countries (fewer than 92), net of the
influence of family planning, a situation that could be a result
of the lower social insurance program experience of these countries. But as Kelly, Cutright, and Hittle (1976) note, such
programs take a long time to affect levels of fertility. Economic
development has a far more pervasive and immediate effect on
fertility. Thus, social insurance programs are not feasible
means for a short-term intervention in fertility.

The state can also legislate the age at marriage, and a higher average age at marriage can lead to lower fertility. The proportion of single women aged fifteen to twenty-four has a negative influence on fertility when included in place of an indicator of women's economic status in the basic model (see Table 5.6, "a" columns). When infant mortality is included in the model ("b" columns), the effects of single women become nonsignificant. When either income inequality or family planning program effort are entered into the equations ("c" and "d" columns), the proportion of single women remains significant and negative. At the same time, women's share of education becomes nonsignificant. Because of the lower number of cases, these results should be interpreted cautiously.[10] The results do indicate, however, that an increase in the proportion of single women has a significant negative effect on fertility, net of the effects of family planning, income inequality, and women's education, but not net of infant mortality. Thus, in countries where women marry at a later age, lower fertility rates prevail (Dixon 1975); this relationship is affected by the presence of higher levels of infant mortality.

A final consideration is the influence of organizational and political status-of-women indicators on the determination of fertility behavior. The effects of women's groups, integration of women in government, women's political rights, and experience with suffrage are examined in the basic regression equation. Of these four indicators and in analyses not reported here, only suffrage experience is significant and has a negative influence on fertility, net of the level of infant mortality. These effects disappear when controlling for either income inequality or family planning effort (Ward 1982). Thus, economic factors, in general, and the educational and economic status of women, in particular, are more important than women's organizational and political status.

In summary, the relationships between investment/ dependency, the status of women, development, and intervening variables are as follows: The positive effects of investment and dependency on fertility are reduced by intervening factors, such as infant mortality and income inequality, that exert pressures toward higher fertility. In this context, development and the economic status of women depress fertility behavior. After controlling for investment/development and income inequality, however, the development effects are strong but lowered, and some of the previously observed negative relationships between women's share of education, economic resources, and fertility are reduced to nonsignificance. At the same time,

TABLE 5.6

OLS Estimates of the Influence of Investment/Dependency, Single Women Aged 15-24, and Intervening Mechanisms on Fertility, 1975

Variables	Unstandardized and Standardized Coefficients							
	a	b	a	b	c	d	c	d
COM CON[†]	17.90** (.20)	10.74 (.12)			-2.39 (-.04)	10.51 (.12)		
MNC INV EXT[†]			12.39** (.19)	7.50* (.11)			-.22 (-.01)	9.91** (.15)
KWHC[†]	-739.24** (-.47)	-596.92** (-.48)	-799.07** (-.65)	-660.31** (.54)	-249.97* (-.24)	-638.76** (-.53)	-178.65 (-.16)	-691.90** (-.56)
FEM TERT ED[‡]	-15.15 (-.07)	-14.22 (-.08)	-15.31 (-.08)	-12.05 (-.07)	-16.28 (-.16)	-7.18 (-.04)	-8.96 (-.08)	-9.49 (-.05)
% SING WOM[§]	-26.60** (-.33)	-14.53 (-.11)	-26.95** (-.21)	-17.86 (-.14)	-23.01* (-.28)	-30.89** (-.23)	-28.75** (-.36)	-28.01** (-.20)
FAM PLAN[§]					-73.53** (.46)		-72.60** (-.47)	
GINI[†]						52.85** (.28)		47.22** (.26)
INF MORT[‡]		10.74** (.28)		8.95** (.24)				
Intercept	10371.76	8153.40	11224.31	9055.69	9311.7	7545.09	8895.67	8297.21
R²	.79	.82	.79	.83	.66	.86	.71	.87
N	58	55	67	61	35	45	39	52

[†] Measured circa 1965.

[‡] Measured circa 1970.

[§] Family planning scores are available only for developing countries.

*$p < .10$.

**$p < .05$.

Note: Variables are defined in Table 5.1. "a" columns depict the basic model; "b" columns include infant mortality; "c" columns include family planning; "d" columns include GINI.

in a restricted sample of developing countries, family planning program efforts have strong negative effects on fertility, net of the influence of either income inequality or infant mortality. (The latter variable becomes nonsignificant.)

If the effects of investment and dependency are to lower the economic status of women relative to men and to raise income inequality and possibly infant mortality, family planning programs may become less effective. Furthermore, the antinatalist effects of changes in foreign investment, in particular, for the reduction of fertility become negligible under these socioeconomic conditions. Thus, although family planning programs are a prudent investment, in the long run, additional intervention into the processes of foreign investment and trade dependency and the pursuant negative effects of underdevelopment on the economic status of women can only strengthen the effects of development and the economic status of women on reducing fertility. Other research also indicates that family planning programs are more effective when women have access to alternative economic resources (Youssef 1979).

In regard to other intervening variables, the state, through the provision of social insurance and family planning programs, has negative effects on fertility. The proportion of single women also exerts negative effects. Last, other organizational and political status-of-women variables exhibit nonsignificant effects on fertility. Thus, from these results, a final model of fertility should include measures of development, infant mortality, family planning, and income inequality. Other variables that should be included are measures of investment and dependency, which are suggested as having indirect effects on fertility, and the status of women in education and the labor force variables, which have small but significant negative effects on fertility.

DISCUSSION

From these findings, we infer that investment and dependency have only small indirect effects on fertility behavior through the intervening mechanisms of infant mortality, income inequality, and the economic status of women. At the same time, development has a strong but reduced negative effect on fertility when the intervening variables are controlled; the negative effects of family planning program effort and state programs are also indicated. In this section I will examine these findings in the context of the previous literature. Then

I will delineate the implications of these findings for possible interventions to lower fertility behavior.

World-System and Inequality

Tilly (1978) has argued that the international patterns of fertility are related more to patterns of international economic relationships than to internal nation-state phenomena. Likewise, Repetto (1979) has found that income inequality among nations is an equally important or potentially greater determinant of fertility than economic development. As one consequence of investment and dependency is income inequality, the small indirect effects of investment and dependency through income inequality exhibited in this research only partially support the earlier arguments of Tilly and Repetto, because development has a stronger effect on fertility than does income inequality. Additionally, if, in the course of international economic relationships, investment/dependency and income inequality are determinants of infant mortality, the pattern of small indirect effects of investment and dependency through infant mortality makes sense as well. In other words, nations experiencing underdevelopment are less likely to provide good prenatal, early child health, and nutritional care, leading to higher infant mortality rates. In particular, the relationship between commodity concentration and infant mortality found in this research merits further attention.

The effects of classical dependency and dependent development (the latter measured by foreign investment) are mediated by internal nation-state phenomena. The findings of small indirect positive effects of investment and dependency on fertility are somewhat different than those results found for Latin America by Hout (1980, 1981), who reported positive and curvilinear effects of trade dependency on fertility.

The methodological differences between Hout's and this research may explain the dissimilar findings. First, Hout utilized pooled cross-sections in time series analysis for Latin America, in contrast to the cross-sectional and cross-national analyses used in this research. Second, no measures of income inequality or the status of women were used in his analysis. The differences among these two sets of findings could be a function of analysis techniques, region, or different model specification.

Hout's arguments that dependency must decline before development affects fertility, although not statistically supported

by my research, require some attention because of the positive
effects of income inequality and infant mortality on fertility,
net of economic development, found in my research. Heightened
income inequality and pursuant social consequences such as
infant mortality brought about by both classical dependency
and dependent development can lower the negative effects of
development on fertility. In essence, an economic population
cycle may evolve: The economic structures produced by investment and dependency generate inadequate economic and social
resources for the population, thereby leading to income inequality,
lowered relative economic development, and disincentives for
the reduction of fertility. With increasing levels of population
growth, the distribution of economic and social resources relative
to the population is further hindered. As development is a
major determinant of fertility, one point of intervention within
this cycle is changes in the relationships among dependency/
investment, economic development, and income inequality,
which can diminish the effects of development on fertility. For
example, if one consequence of investment and dependency is
lowered relative rates of economic growth, changes in investment
and dependency as proposed in the New International Economic
Order (Ul Haq 1979) may increase the influence of economic
development on fertility. Alternatively, more equitable distribu-
tions of income should result in the reduction of fertility.
Another point of intervention is the economic status of women,
which is lowered by investment and dependency relationships.

Status of Women

Improvement in women's economic status has a small negative
influence on fertility, net of most factors, with the exception
of some of the equations that include income inequality. The
negative effects of women's share of education diminish when
infant mortality is controlled in the regression equations.
Furthermore, as noted in chapter 4, women's economic status
is adversely affected by investment and dependency relations.
Hence, part of the reason the effects of women's economic status
on fertility are small is because of the effects of investment
and dependency on the relationship between women's economic
status and fertility. First, as noted in chapter 4, with increased
levels of investment and dependency, women have lowered access
to the new economic resources generated, particularly industrial
jobs. Second, as noted by other researchers, women's traditional
modes of economic livelihood are disrupted by investment and

dependency. Owing to these two effects, previous negative relationships between women's work and fertility found in developed countries may become limited or negligible as many women in developing countries have less access to the formal labor force and are relegated to the informal sector. As a result, the levels of fertility may remain high compared with those found in developed countries. Thus, the limited effects of women's economic status, net of investment and dependency, suggest a partial explanation for the inconsistent cross-national findings between women's economic status and fertility noted by Kupinsky (1977a) and Standing (1978). These researchers did not control for investment and dependency.

These macro relationships may affect fertility decision-making at the micro level, because, in Coale's (1973) terms, many women may be unable consciously to choose fertility reduction or may find such reduction economically disadvantageous. Under the conditions of underdevelopment, women's power or control over fertility is lowered within the family because of women's lowered access to the new economic resources relative to men's; also, the value of children remains high, as a source of either income or social status (Hass 1972; Dixon 1975; Caldwell 1976; Newland 1977; ICRW 1980b). Thus, children are one means for women to generate leverage over their environment, and the care of children is easily combined with participation within the informal labor market (Newland 1977; Youssef 1979; Safilios-Rothschild 1982). Therefore, in the context of developing countries, traditional models of fertility behavior are incomplete. As Youssef notes:

> The premise for this particular model [human capital or traditional models of fertility] bears some relevance to conditions characterizing a tiny minority of upper and middle class women whose education gives them access to stimulating, creative, and ego-fulfilling jobs that offer satisfaction and rewarding alternatives to childbearing. The explanatory variables lose much of their appeal in interpreting the employment fertility relationship among low-income women (1979, p. 16).

Women's Education

The small or inconsistent effects of women's share of tertiary education indicate that women's access to tertiary education has only a limited negative influence on fertility. This limited influence is congruent with research cited previously, which has noted that the negative relationship between education and fertility in developing countries is lowered if educated women are unable to find work commensurate with their education (Dixon 1975). This relationship is weakened further when sons are educated first and are the family members most likely to find employment. The negative effect of education on fertility is unlikely to increase because parents are unwilling to invest in their daughters' continued education. As a consequence, women, through lesser access to education, will lack exposure to new ideas, values, and education, which in turn affect fertility behavior (Dixon 1975). Finally, given the low level of formal employment opportunities for women in developing countries and low levels of literacy, other social factors such as infant mortality can intervene in the education and fertility relationship.

Organizational and Political Status

The negligible effects of women's organizational and political status on fertility may be due to either poor measures of these variables or a lack of direct effects on fertility. Obviously, the organizational measure may inadequately represent the extent and nature of women's organizational activities, since information about particular family planning and employment programs sponsored by such organizations is unavailable. Other researchers have demonstrated that, within individual nation-states, women's organizations are good sites for education, employment, and family planning programs (Bruce 1976; Dixon 1978b). When better data on women's organizations and programs are available, the actual cross-national effectiveness of women's organizations in the reduction of fertility needs further examination. The negligible effects of the integration of women within government and women's political status indicate that these factors have yet to demonstrate direct negative effects on women's fertility. Evidence from developing nation-states indicates that women still lack access to policy-making positions (Chaney 1973; Newland 1979). Further, equal rights and pay legislation is often inaccessible and inapplicable to the realities of most women's work lives (Newland 1979; Mazumdar 1979; Chaney and Schmink 1980). Hence, women's organizational and political status in developing countries has little direct bearing on the determination of fertility.

Family Planning Program Effort

The negative effects of family planning on fertility need to be evaluated in light of dependency, investment, under-development, and the status of women, as discussed in the preceding sections. First, these negative family planning effects are found for a sample limited to developing countries, in contrast to the small but more economically diverse sample used in the infant mortality and income inequality equations. Thus, these effects could be biased upwards, as the overall variation in investment and dependency is limited and the relationships among investment, dependency, and fertility are reduced. Second, as argued previously, income inequality and, in particular, infant mortality provide underlying pressures toward higher fertility.[11] If developing nations rely only on technological solutions or family planning programs, these pro-grams can be undermined by the positive effects of income inequality and infant mortality. Third, these programs could be more effective if women had greater control over fertility behavior because of increased access to economic resources (Youssef 1979).

Family planning programs are important for the reduction of fertility, but the results of this study suggest that these programs should be implemented as part of a diverse strategy for fertility reduction. As Coale (1973) notes, the provision of family planning is only one of three factors necessary to bring about a fertility decline. (The other factors are conscious choices over fertility and a perception that the reduction of fertility is socially and economically advantageous.) By con-centrating solely on family planning programs, researchers ignore other possible interventions that could have more benefits besides fertility reduction: changes in investment/dependency relationships and improvement in the economic status of women. These factors can strengthen development efforts while contribut-ing to lower fertility rates.

One possible site for the coordination of family planning efforts and interventions in investment, dependency, and the status of women is the state, which can provide social insurance programs that lower the value of children (Hohm 1975). Ramirez and Thomas (1981) argue that weak states can evolve into stronger states through interaction with the international economy and developed nation-states, thereby counteracting some of the negative consequences of investment and dependency on state strength. Further, centrally planned economies have higher levels of female economic participation. The state, therefore, can mitigate the effects of investment/dependency while incorporating women more fully into the economy. With the judicious provision of family planning services, fertility could be reduced in this particular socioeconomic setting.

In conclusion, the determination of fertility behavior cross-nationally is complex. To build on the previous theoretical and empirical work on the effects of development, family planning, and infant mortality on fertility, the small effects of the world-system, income inequality, and the status of women found in this research merit further investigation and incorporation into theories of the world-system and fertility.

NOTES

1. These tests are performed by first estimating the following equation:

$$\text{fertility} = a + b \text{ INV/DEP} + b \text{ KWHC} =$$
$$b \text{ FEM SHA LF} + b \text{ FEM TERT ED} + e$$

Interaction terms are constructed by multiplying an investment/dependency indicator by the kilowatt hours per capita indicator (INV/DEP × KWHC). The curvilinear relationship between development and fertility is represented by a squared development term (KWHC^2). Then these terms are entered into the first equation by separate investment and dependency indicators. The increment in R^2 with the addition of these terms is not significant at the $\underline{p} < .05$ level, and the individual interaction or squared terms also are not significant, with the exception of one equation. This equation was not interpretable due to multicollinearity. As will be noted later in the discussion section, the reasons for the nonsignificant effects of the interaction or curvilinear terms may be the use of a cross-national versus a regional sample and differential model specification.

2. A lagged dependent variable is not used due to the high correlation between the total fertility rate in 1968 and that in 1975 ($r = .96$); thus, the range of variation in fertility in 1975 is examined. A measure of state strength is not included in the basic equation for similar reasons: The correlation between energy usage and the state is $r = .70$. Finally, results are

reported only for significant investment/dependency equations. For example, TNC investment in agriculture and manufacturing and the change in commodity concentration and the foreign trade structure have nonsignificant effects on fertility behavior.

3. Given the past research on the efforts of centrally planned economies, the effects of such economies on fertility behavior are of interest. As in the analyses reported in chapter 4, the dummy variable for centrally planned economies was entered into the equations; although the results for the other independent variables remain the same, the dummy variable has a positive effect on fertility when included in the equation for women's share of the labor force and participation and a negative effect for the other economic status-of-women equations. Thus, centrally planned economies have higher levels of fertility than would be expected for countries with high levels of women's participation. When other intervening variables are controlled, however, the effects of the dummy variable are reduced to nonsignificance.

4. This particular research strategy is used to examine the separate effects of the same intervening variables because of the different numbers of cases for which data are available on all three variables.

5. In equations using the other economic status-of-women variables, the influence of women's economic status is reduced or becomes nonsignificant.

6. Separate analyses indicate that the level of infant mortality is related to dependency and investment. Infant mortality in 1968 is regressed on indicators of investment and dependency circa 1965 while controlling for the level of development in 1965. Of the investment and dependency indicators, commodity concentration and TNC investment in extraction have significant and positive effects on the level of infant mortality. The standardized coefficients for the commodity concentration equation are .17 for commodity concentration and -.72 for KWHC; the similar coefficients for the extraction equations are .22 for TNC extraction and -.80 for KWHC. Thus, although the level of energy usage is a stronger determinant of infant mortality, these measures of investment and dependency have a positive influence on infant mortality, suggesting the presence of indirect effects of investment and dependency on fertility through infant mortality.

7. After controlling for income inequality, the effects of women's labor-force participation and women's share of sectors become nonsignificant.

8. Although the number of cases in the equations that include both income inequality and infant mortality is lower than in other equations, the countries represented in the equations are more diverse in terms of investment and level of development than the more homogeneous sample of developing countries for which the Mauldin-Berelson family planning program effort variable is available.

9. If all three variables are included in the equation, the number of cases becomes prohibitively low.

10. Also due to the low number of cases, the effect of the proportion of single women net of the combined effects of the intervening variables remains untested.

11. Still other researchers have argued that high levels of fertility lead to high levels of infant mortality (Scrimshaw 1978). Under these conditions, children born later receive less attention and care than earlier children; therefore, there is a potential for high levels of infant mortality at high levels of fertility. At the same time, infant mortality could be related to fertility through the increased socioeconomic value of children. In societies with high infant mortality, the deaths of children may result in the replacement of at least some of the children. Hence, earlier levels of infant mortality may affect the later levels of fertility. Either way, these relationships between infant mortality and fertility merit further attention at the aggregate level.

6
Summary and Discussion

In this chapter, the original arguments about the influence of the world system on the status of women and, in turn, the influence of these two phenomena on fertility behavior are examined in light of regression analyses presented in chapters 4 and 5. First, the hypotheses on the status of women are reviewed followed by the results from the chapter on women's share of economic resources and fertility. Then the hypotheses and the findings for fertility from chapter 5 are discussed in a similar manner. Second, specification and measurement issues are examined with attention to the limitations on the findings posed by problems with cross-sectional designs and data on the status of women. Finally, implications and directions for theory, research, and policy on the world system, women in development, and fertility are outlined.

SUMMARY OF THEORETICAL ARGUMENTS AND RESULTS

Economic Status of Women

In chapter 2, the world system, through the intrusion of foreign investment and trade dependency, was hypothesized to have a negative effect on women's share of economic resources. Second, specific intervening mechanisms—the labor force relative to the total population, the state, and urbanization—and specific distributional factors—bureaucratization, power sharing with experts, and unions—were hypothesized to mediate the effects of investment and dependency. Third, an additional consequence

of world-system relationships, income inequality, was predicted
to have negative effects on women's share of educational and
economic resources. Fourth, variables representing other
facets of women's organizational and political status were control
variables and were expected to have positive effects on women's
share of educational and economic resources.

The predicted relationships between classical dependency
and dependent development and the economic status of women
appear to be supported in this research. Dependency and
investment indicators have direct negative effects on women's
share of the total labor force and participation; certain negative
relationships of both types of dependency are even stronger
when women's shares of the agricultural and industrial sectors
are considered. Of the intervening variables, the effects of
change in the size of the total labor force relative to the adult
population are significant and positive. The size of the service
sector relative to the total labor force has negative effects.[1]

State strength and economic development have only small
and frequently nonsignificant effects on women's economic status
in contrast with the substantial positive effects of centrally
planned economies. Further, power sharing with experts is
indicated as a factor that enhances women's share of the labor
force; income inequality more strongly affects women's share of
industry than women's overall share of the labor force. Finally,
other status-of-women variables such as women's share of
tertiary education have rather small and nonsignificant effects.

In this research, therefore, the linkages between the
world-system and the economic status of women are supported.
Other variables that were previously found to affect women's
status, such as the level of economic development and state
strength, are relatively ineffectual in raising the economic status
of women. This is due, in part, to the economic conditions
brought about by investment and dependency. Additionally,
investment and dependency have negative indirect effects on
women's status through the size of the labor force, service
sector, urbanization, and income inequality. With the meager
structure of economic opportunities, women in developing
countries have limited access to economic resources, particularly,
women's access to industrial and formally recognized agricultural
work. Women's access to the service sector is dependent on
the specific level of economic development.

The effects of these international and intervening economic
relationships on women's large-scale participation in the informal
economic sector are only indicated indirectly because large
numbers of women are unrepresented in the formal labor-force

statistics. Previous research has found that the informal labor markets are a major means of subsistence for women and that investment and dependency have negative effects on women's economic participation, both formal and informal. Under these conditions of underdevelopment generated by classical dependency and dependent development, women relative to men are at a substantial disadvantage in the competition for access to and control over resources.

Fertility Behavior

In chapter 2 the world economic system, through foreign investment and trade dependency, was predicted to have positive direct effects on fertility. Investment and dependency were expected to work indirectly through lowered status of women and heightened income inequality to raise fertility. Economic development and other social setting factors, e.g., infant mortality and family planning, were also predicted to affect fertility. Of particular interest were the relative effects of economic development, status of women, and family planning program efforts on fertility after controlling for investment/dependency, because in past research the status of women and investment/dependency have been rarely included in analyses.

As noted in chapter 5, the small effects of investment and dependency on fertility operate indirectly through infant mortality and income inequality.[2] In this setting, the economic status of women and development have negative effects on fertility. However, the previous negative relationships between women's education, employment, and fertility are lowered or become nonsignificant. The development effects, although diminished, remain among the strongest determinants of fertility. In a smaller group of developing countries, family planning program efforts have a strong negative influence on fertility, net of either income inequality or infant mortality. Even so, the combined effects of income inequality and infant mortality on fertility constitute pressures toward maintaining high levels of fertility. From these analyses, development, family planning, and infant mortality constitute the strongest determinants of fertility. Lesser but significant effects are shown for income inequality, the educational and economic status of women, and investment/dependency.

SPECIFICATION AND MEASUREMENT ISSUES

In this section, I examine the problems posed by the use
of cross-sectional analysis techniques and model specification.
Second, the data on the status of women are reevaluated in
light of the theoretical arguments and the performance of these
variables in regression analysis.

Cross-Sectional Design

The cross-sectional design used in the analyses of women's
economic status and fertility behavior and the interpretation
of these results are subject to bias due to reciprocal relationships. Further, only recursive paths are estimated, a situation
that can lead to possible specification error. The presence of
reciprocal relationships, therefore, can bias the results of the
economic status-of-women and fertility equations, especially if
the economic status-of-women variables have affected income
inequality and if the earlier levels of fertility have affected
women's economic status.

First, although previous research has specified that income
inequality is a determinant of women's share of labor-force
resources, an argument for the opposite relationship is made
in chapter 2. If the true ordering is that women's share of
resources determines income inequality, the model used in this
research is misspecified. Alternatively, if the relationship
between women's economic status and income inequality is
reciprocal, the model could also be misspecified. As income
inequality data are currently available for only one time point,
recently available estimates of income inequality in 1975 can be
used in future analyses to test the potential nonrecursive or
reciprocal relationship between women's economic status and
income inequality.

Second, the issue of the women's labor force and fertility
ordering is a potential threat to the validity of these results.
According to a review of the recent literature, the specific
ordering of this relationship is subject to considerable debate
among scholars (Kupinsky 1977a, 1977b; Standing 1978; Youssef
1979). In past cross-national treatments of this relationship,
for example, Semyonov's (1980) research, the fertility rate at
one point in time has been assumed to affect women's labor-force
participation, but researchers have not explicitly considered
how the earlier structure of economic opportunities for women
generated by international and indigenous economic relationships

affects fertility. Obviously, fertility within a given year affects women's labor-force participation in the same year. Nevertheless, the earlier demand for female labor and women's access to economic resources affect later levels of fertility. In the short run, fertility influences women's share of the labor force (Standing 1978); in the long run, fertility is governed by economic and social conditions (Davis and Blake 1956), of which women's economic status is a major component. Thus, theoretically, the employment-fertility ordering is justified. (For a review of opposing arguments, see Dixon 1978b and Youssef 1982.) An important task for future research, however, is to continue efforts to specify the theoretically fruitful concept of the dialectical relationship between women's work and reproductive roles noted by Sokoloff (1980). The use of this concept in future research may resolve some of the debate over the employment-fertility ordering.

In general, although the cross-sectional design precludes the specific testing of these potential reciprocal relationships and multicollinearity prohibits the inclusion of lagged dependent variables to control for reciprocal bias, specific theoretical guidance and the time-ordering of variables in these analyses should provide better estimates of the determinants of women's economic status and fertility than if the independent and dependent variables were measured at the same point in time. Further, since cross-sectional analyses only represent the influence of the independent variables on the variation across nations in the dependent variable at one point in time, future research might usefully explain the issue of how much change in the dependent variables over time is attributable to changes in the independent variables.

Status of Women Data

Reliability and validity problems are inherent in cross-national data on the status of women; this research is no exception. Specific points of concern include: (1) the strength and explanatory completeness of the empirical relationships estimated from the status-of-women data compared to those of the theoretical relationships formulated in this research; and (2) interpretations relative to the effects of investment and dependency on women in formal and informal labor markets.

In general, the status-of-women data are available for fewer cases and the standards of conceptualization and measurement are much cruder than conventional measures of cross-national phenomena. As a result, missing data are a major problem, especially if list-wise deletion of missing cases is used in analysis. Further, estimates are unstable because of shifting numbers of cases. Finally, the validity of these measures is questionable.

Even so, a moderate amount of congruence between theoretical and empirical relationships is found in this research, suggesting that the investment/dependency, intervening mechanisms, and status-of-women indicators used reflect the presence of the specified theoretical relationships. In other words, investment and dependency account for at least part of the variation in women's share of economic resources.

At the same time, the size of these relationships and the amount of variation explained are disappointingly small in contrast to those of other cross-national research. Two possibly interrelated explanations for the size of the relationships are (1) that the number of cases is larger and (2) that formal labor-force statistics are representative of only a small minority of women in developing nations. First, past cross-national research on women's share of the labor force has utilized more homogeneous samples of either several regions or, on the average, 60 countries (Youssef 1974; Weiss, Ramirez, and Tracy 1976; Semyonov 1980). In this sample, there are a much larger number of cases, thereby increasing the heterogeneity of the sample. Furthermore, examining the correlations generated in past research reveals that the correlations between socioeconomic phenomena and women's share of the labor force are smaller than the correlations observed for other cross-national relationships, such as those between economic development and income inequality. However, the sizes of the empirical relationships found in this research are similar to those observed in other research on women's share of the labor force.

As to the second explanation of these results, the vagaries of cross-national measurement of women's economic participation and the location of many women within informal labor markets may be responsible for the small relationships found in this research. Researchers have noted that women's participation in economic activities is underrepresented in numerous countries, owing to incomplete reporting systems, official definitions of female activities, and misleading reports by the women themselves (Youssef 1979; ICRW 1980a, 1980b; Dixon 1982). Further, only a minority of women from developing countries may actually be represented by the labor-force estimates used in this research. Many women are participating in the informal labor market—a situation indirectly measured by International Labor Office estimates. The size of this labor market, as noted previously, is quite large, but no cross-national estimates exist for analysis. To the extent that women are located in this informal labor market, the empirical results for women's formal participation are attenuated.

Until better data on women's economic activity are available, the precision and accuracy of research using these data are reduced, and the results should be interpreted with caution. The short-run solution to this problem, however, is to continue research at the cross-national level and to supplement cross-national data with case and women's time-use studies from individual nation-states and regions (Dixon 1982). Since, despite measurement problems, the theoretical relationships outlined in this research are tentatively supported, these findings have implications for world-system and women in development research and provide directions for future theoretical, empirical, and research efforts.

IMPLICATIONS FOR THEORY, RESEARCH, AND POLICY

This book has drawn together three bodies of literature. Hence, the implications of this research are applicable to theory and research on the world economic system, women in development, and fertility and for policy in the areas of women in development and fertility.

World Economic System

The findings suggest that previous theoretical formulations on the processes and consequences of the world-system are incomplete, since they neglect the role of women. More specifically, they omit consideration of the lowered economic status of women under the processes of classical dependency and dependent development. Additional theoretical formulations of women's role within the world-system are needed. The significant negative effects of investment and dependency on the economic status of women suggest that we cannot assume that the processes of the world-system affect women and men in the same manner. For example, excessive service-sector growth or urbanization are suggested as having negative effects on women's access to resources relative to men's (Ward in press). Some labor-force consequences of investment and dependency

affect women and men differently in terms of access to formal
employment and to the agricultural and industrial sectors.
Similarly, women in industries are more negatively affected
than men by integration in the global assembly line of transnational corporations. Hence, the effects of the consequences
of the world-system need to be systematically reexamined in
light of these sex-specific effects or consequences.

Women's reduced share of economic resources under investment and dependency can also be interpreted as representing
a situation (as noted in chapter 2) where through the processes
of the world economic system and patriarchial relations, men
have gained an external sphere of control over economic resources in the public domain (Sanday 1974). These findings
and interpretations do not indicate that all men have access to
economic resources or employment during the processes induced
by investment and dependency. Instead, I propose that men
as a group have disproportionate access to and control over
such resources generated by the international division of labor.
The sex differences in access are a major hardship for women
who are expected socially to be economically self-sufficient
following migration, disruption of family structures, and growth
of female-headed households that have low incomes. For these
women, the lack of access to economic resources means a constant struggle for survival—a struggle where many women have
no choice with regard to economic activity. Yet through the
marginalization of women from production under international
economic and patriarchial relationships, many women and their
families are relegated to continued poverty amidst underdevelopment. The problems of women in development, therefore, result
in part from the international economic relationships and the
limited structure of opportunities generated by investment and
dependency and controlled by men or male elites rather than
problems related only to ideological or cultural constraints.
Obviously, other important determinants of women's economic
status within the world-system remain to be identified.

Further, the potential feedback effects of women's status
on economic growth and income inequality need to be reconsidered.
Other researchers have proposed that women's informal labor
market participation constitutes a hidden prop to development
that is being disrupted by the negative consequences of development on women (Boulding 1977). This argument and the findings
of the negative effects of investment/dependency on women's
share of economic resources suggest that women's lowered status
may contribute to the components of underdevelopment: lowered
relative rates of economic growth and heightened income inequal-

ity. Thus, if women's contribution to development is disrupted and if women have diminished access to economic resources, economic growth may be harmed, and income inequality may increase. The declining status of women as a determinant of development and income inequality needs further theoretical work.

Women in Development

The processes of the world-system need to be incorporated into theoretical frameworks or paradigms on women in develop-ment, such as those formulated by Blumberg (1978) and Sanday (1974, 1981). Frequently, these frameworks have specified the conditions under which women have declining access to economic resources without noting the potential effects of international economic relationships on women's status across or within individ-ual nation-states. The significant cross-national effects of investment and dependency on women's economic status suggest that these previous theoretical frameworks are incomplete. The problems of women in development may in fact be related to the particular forms that development (or underdevelopment) takes after contact with foreign investment and dependency, yet these factors are notably missing in cross-national theories of women in development. The results do support the previous contention that development (broadly defined) has a negative influence on women's economic status, but the effects of investment and dependency on women's status appear to be one of the reasons that development has had a negative influence on women's eco-nomic status in developing countries.

At the same time, these results fail to support theoretical predictions that women's status can be improved by further incorporation into the prevailing setting of development in developing countries (Boserup 1970; Tinker 1976). Because of the negative effects of investment and dependency on eco-nomic growth and women's access to formal economic resources, women in developing countries may find further access to the labor force difficult, as in these circumstances women are fre-quently marginalized from production. Thus, the theoretical problem is not that women have not been integrated into develop-ment, but rather that due to the certain economic patterns brought about by investment and dependency, women and men have different access to resources generated by investment and dependency (see, for example, the studies in Nash and Fernández-Kelly 1983). In the long run, this difference in access may be perpetuated in the peripheral nations by the world capitalist system, in contrast with the experience of the core nations, where women have been gradually brought back into production and the formal labor force.

Research at the macro level in the area of women in development needs to include indicators of investment and dependency in empirical analyses. Otherwise, the effects of other variables, such as economic development, on women's economic status are likely to be overestimated. At the same time, the inclusion of investment and dependency variables only partially explains the variation in women's access to economic resources. This partial explanation could stem from the influence of other unspecified factors at the international and nation-state level or to data that may only reflect the formal economic participation of a minority of women in developing countries. The significant effects of intervening factors such as income inequality or power sharing with experts suggest that factors within particular nations also affect women's access to economic resources. Hence, researchers on women in development must further specify omitted factors. Additionally, until cross-national data on women's informal-sector participation are available or generated from individual nation-state research, the cross-national data on women's formal participation should be used with caution.

At the micro level, researchers need to specify how investment and dependency within individual nation-states affect women's access to resources such as factory or agricultural production. More regional and local studies informed by a dependency or world-system perspective are needed, like the studies by Deere and Leon de Leal (1981) in Colombia and Peru, Fernández-Kelly (1983) in Mexico, and Bossen (1984) in Guatemala. Further, the cross-national effects of investment and dependency on women's participation in the informal labor markets can only be inferred from micro research. In order to generate cross-national data on these markets, more research is needed on how specific forms of investment and trade dependency affect women's informal labor market participation within individual nation-states. Last, the influence of investment and dependency on the effectiveness of programs to incorporate women into the formal labor force requires additional research. For example, development programs that promote women's production of goods or provision of services may unsuccessfully compete with the goods or services of transnational corporations.

The policy implications from this research are relevant for efforts to improve the status of women during development. This research suggests that foreign investment and trade dependency have negative effects on women's access to the total labor force and the agricultural and industrial sectors. In order to integrate women into the formal labor force, policy-makers should examine the effects of traditional investment policies and programs on women's access to the labor force, as in the past these policies and programs appear to have placed women at a competitive disadvantage with men in the labor force.

Likewise, transnational corporation investment appears to lower women's overall access to the labor force and to the industrial sector. As a consequence, TNC investment should be carefully structured to provide a maximum of long-term and productive employment for women that will provide income for both women and the nation-state. As Fernández-Kelly (1983) noted, however, employment in the TNC plants increases the vulnerability of women.

The International Center for Research on Women (1980b) recommends that development planners implement policies that regulate the TNCs' employment of women, provide long-term employment alternatives for women, and oversee the employment and training of women in TNC plants (1980b, pp. 90-92). First, nation-states need to guarantee humane treatment and opportunities to workers involved in TNC employment while working with other nation-states in the region to prevent runaway plants and hazardous working conditions. Second, governments should encourage the growth of labor-intensive production for import substitution so that capital generated by such plants stays in the country and dependence on foreign products is reduced. Third, women's employment opportunities in TNC plants should be stabilized through equal opportunity practices, notices of layoff, and compensation for unemployed TNC workers. Fourth, women workers should be allowed access to union organization and protective legislation by the TNCs and the state governments. Finally, women should be involved in all facets of production (including management) so that they will be able to acquire skills that can be transferred to other employment settings. Ideally, with these changes in policies and employment, developing countries can incorporate women into the labor force with minimum costs for development and maximum benefits for development efforts.

Fertility

These findings indicate that, first, in contrast to earlier theoretical arguments, the previous relationships between eco-

nomic development and fertility are only slightly reduced if
the influence of the world economic system and pursuant income
inequality are controlled. Second, the economic status of women
has a small independent and negative influence on fertility that
remains after controlling for other social phenomena, such as
infant mortality and family planning. The influence of women's
economic status on fertility, however, is reduced when
investment/dependency and income inequality are controlled,
which could account for the previous contradictory findings on
the relationships between economic development, women's
employment, and fertility, which at various times have been
negative, positive, or negligible (Kupinsky 1977a; Standing
1978). The theoretical importance of these findings on the
relative influence of economic development and the status of
women is that these variables can have independent effects on
fertility behavior, but the influence of the status of women is
linked to the structure of economic opportunities that occur
with investment and dependency.

Family Planning

    The influence of family planning efforts on fertility net
of investment, dependency, and other specified variables is
striking in this research. Yet when this influence is considered
in light of the relationships among investment, dependency,
income inequality, infant mortality, and the status of women,
these variables obviously can impede the rapid and continued
reduction of fertility, despite family planning efforts. For
example, with women's lowered status under investment and
dependency, women may be less likely to gain leverage over
their environment and be unable to make conscious choices
about fertility reduction. Meanwhile, children remain economically
and socially advantageous. In a similar manner, the positive
effects of infant mortality and income inequality provide barriers
against the reduction of fertility. In conjunction with the relative
status of women and limited economic opportunities for the population as a whole, these factors are possible disincentives to
limit the number of children and to utilize family planning programs.
    From these concerns, family planning programs can be
more effective if instituted with changes in the patterns of
investment/dependency, underdevelopment, and the status of
women. First, if the effects of investment and dependency are
lowered relative rates of economic growth and underdevelopment
for developing countries compared with developed countries,
economic development and family planning programs can have

greater effects on fertility through changes in investment/ dependency that bring economic growth, development, and resources to the entire population. A number of researchers have argued that the implementation and effectiveness of family planning programs are related to the socioeconomic structures of countries, thereby questioning the uncritical advocacy of family planning programs. Demeny (1979) has argued that in many countries these socioeconomic structures led to a decline in fertility that in turn generated the implementation of family planning programs. Likewise, Hernandez (1981) has noted that the effectiveness of family planning programs is affected by the antecedent socioeconomic conditions. Thus, advocating the proliferation of family planning programs without undertaking changes in the underlying socioeconomic conditions is a questionable course. For example, family planning programs that are mandated by investment packages are likely to be less than effective owing to underdevelopment generated by such packages.

Second, changes in the educational and economic status of women are theoretically important for the effectiveness of family planning programs. Otherwise, as Elu de Lenero (1980) and other researchers have noted, women will continue to receive contradictory messages about fertility behavior. On the one hand, through family planning programs, women are told to limit their families; on the other hand, owing to investment/ dependency, women are marginalized from economic production and are relegated to childbearing as a means of status—a contradiction rarely noted in the family planning literature.

Thus, intervention in the processes that lower women's economic status can enhance efforts to bring about development and to lower fertility. The incorporation of women into formal economic activities is predicted to generate new income for development efforts and to enable poor women to more adequately support their families. As Youssef (1979) argues, greater employment of women is important as an intervention to increase the economic opportunities of poor women and development efforts rather than merely as an intervention to reduce fertility. In this sense, the goal is to increase women's economic opportunities instead of merely to utilize women's work as a means to lower fertility. For example, female heads of households need employment, yet these women (who are the poorest of the poor) are frequently denied access to education, employment, housing, and family planning programs (Buvinic, Youssef, and Von Elm 1978). Therefore, if the structure of economic opportunities for women is indeed a determinant of fertility, greater incorporation into formal economic structures could enable women to gain control over the determination of their fertility (Youssef 1979).[3]

Yet this intervention or incorporation of women can be ineffectual if such intervention is undertaken solely to reduce fertility without recognition of the disruptive influence of investment and dependency on women's share of economic resources. An increase in women's employment opportunities would be created in a context of changes in investment and dependency relationships that aid development efforts. Increased employment of women in, for example, transnational microchip plants or offshore sourcing (that is, the partial production of exports for developed countries through factories in developing countries) is an inadequate solution because these jobs are unstable and provide nontransferable training. In addition, the revenues generated by such investments generally flow out of the country. Instead, women can be incorporated in production efforts that involve labor-intensive production for the indigenous economy and enhance efforts to bring about development and lower fertility (for example, see Carr 1978; Dixon 1978b; Youssef 1979).

Patterns of fertility behavior, therefore, must be further interpreted in the context of investment/dependency, the structure of economic opportunities for women, and the additional effects of women's formal employment on fertility. Given the strong effects of family planning and development, these results suggest that theories on the reduction of fertility should incorporate expansion of family planning programs and changes in the patterns of economic development, underdevelopment, infant mortality, income inequality, and the status of women.

Likewise, three directions for fertility research can be derived from these analyses. First, as the effects of family planning net of the above factors were evaluated in a small group of developing countries, the results suggest that more research is needed on the relative effects of development, family planning, and investment/dependency on fertility in a more diverse group of countries. Second, the educational and economic status-of-women variables have independent effects on fertility that are unrepresented by indicators of economic development. For example, past research frequently has used economic development as a proxy variable to represent the status of women (Mauldin and Berelson 1978). Yet the independent influence of women's status on fertility suggests that analyses that omit these factors are likely to overstate the effects of development and other determinants of fertility. Finally, these results indicate that the structure of economic opportunities for women does have an effect on fertility. More research on this relationship, however, needs to be undertaken where the opposite side of this dialectical relationship (between productive and reproductive roles) or the relative effects of fertility on women's access to economic resources are examined and/or controlled.

From the above, policy-makers in the area of fertility should take steps to rectify conditions that may undercut the influence of economic development and family planning programs on fertility, such as higher levels of infant mortality and the lowered status of women under development. Likewise, investment and dependency programs that lower rates of economic growth, raise income inequality, and thereby impede economic development may also diminish the effects of economic development on lowering the value of children. In other words, a diverse strategy involving development, family planning programs, and changes in dependency, infant mortality, income inequality, and the status of women is suggested by this research.

NOTES

1. The substantial correlations between the size of the total labor force relative to the population and women's share of the labor force suggest problems with ratio variables where there are common denominators or numerators. This is also a problem with the size of the service sector relative to the total labor force. As a consequence, these relationships could be overstated. According to theory, however, the size of the relationships is expected to be high, where the relative size of the labor force is predicted to be a major determinant of women's share of the labor force. Thus, the commonality of terms is justified by theoretical considerations.

2. As noted in chapter 5 and in note 6 of that chapter, commodity concentration and transnational investment in extraction have positive effects on infant mortality, net of the effects of development. Further, past research has demonstrated that investment and dependency have positive effects on the level of income inequality, net of the effects of development and other factors (Chase-Dunn 1975; Bornschier and Ballmer-Cao 1979).

3. Another basis for action is intervention(s) that increase both women's status and their power. Women's status is societal in nature, but women's power is "women's ability to influence and control at the interpersonal level" (Safilios-Rothschild 1982, p. 117). The determinants of women's power

in the household therefore are also related to decisions over fertility. (See Safilios-Rothschild 1982 for an elaboration of this micro perspective.) Hence, factors that increase women's power can enhance women's ability to control their reproduction.

COUNTRIES USED IN ANALYSES OF ECONOMIC STATUS OF WOMEN

Women's Share of the Labor Force, Economic Sectors, and Participation

Country	TRSTR	CMCON	ΔTRS	ΔFDI	ΔCOM	GINI
Afghanistan	—	x[a]	—	x	x	—
Albania	—	—	—	—	—	—
Algeria	x	x	—	x	x	—
Angola	—	—	—	x	—	—
Argentina	x	x	x	x	x	x
Australia	x	x	x	x	x	x
Austria	x	x	x	x	x	x
Belgium	x	x	x	x	x	—
Benin	x	x	x	x	x	x
Bolivia	—	x	—	x	—	x
Brazil	x	x	x	x	x	x
Bulgaria	—	—	—	—	—	x
Burma	x	x	x	x	x	x
Burundi	—	—	—	x	—	—
Central African Republic	x	—	x	x	—	—
Cambodia	x	x	x	x	—	—
Cameroon	x	—	x	x	—	—
Canada	x	—	x	x	—	x
Chile	x	x	x	x	x	x
Colombia	x	x	x	x	x	x
Costa Rica	x	x	x	x	x	x
Czechoslovakia	x	x	x	—	x	x
Denmark	x	x	x	x	x	x
Dominican Republic	—	x	—	x	x	—
Ecuador	—	x	—	x	—	x
El Salvador	x	x	x	x	x	x
Ethiopia	x	x	x	x	x	—
Egypt	x	x	x	x	x	x
Finland	x	x	x	x	x	x
France	x	x	x	x	x	x
German Democratic Republic	—	—	—	—	—	x

(continued)

Country	TRSTR	CMCON	ΔTRS	ΔFDI	ΔCOM	GINI
German Federal Republic	x	x	x	x	x	x
Ghana	x	x	x	x	x	x
Greece	x	x	x	x	x	x
Guatemala	x	x	x	x	x	—
Guinea	—	—	—	x	—	—
Hong Kong	x	—	x	x	—	x
Hungary	x	x	x	—	x	x
India	x	x	x	x	x	x
Indonesia	x	x	x	x	x	—
Iran	x	x	x	x	x	—
Iraq	—	x	—	x	x	x
Ireland	x	x	x	x	x	—
Israel	x	x	x	x	x	—
Italy	x	x	x	x	x	x
Ivory Coast	x	x	x	x	x	x
Jamaica	x	—	x	x	—	x
Japan	x	x	x	x	x	x
Jordan	x	x	x	x	—	—
Kenya	x	—	x	x	—	x
Laos	x	—	x	x	—	—
Lebanon	—	—	—	x	—	x
Liberia	x	x	x	x	x	—
Libya	x	x	x	x	x	—
Madagascar	x	x	x	x	x	x
Malawi	x	x	x	x	x	x
Malaysia	x	—	x	x	—	x
Mali	x	—	x	x	—	—
Mexico	x	x	x	x	—	x
Morocco	x	x	x	x	x	x
Mozambique	—	—	—	x	—	—
Netherlands	x	x	x	x	x	x
Nicaragua	x	x	x	x	x	—
Nigeria	x	x	x	x	x	x
Norway	x	x	x	x	x	x
New Zealand	x	x	x	x	x	x
Pakistan	x	x	x	x	x	x
Panama	x	x	x	x	—	x
Paraguay	—	x	—	x	x	—
Peru	x	x	x	x	—	x
Philippines	x	x	x	x	x	x

Country	TRSTR	CMCON	ΔTRS	ΔFDI	ΔCOM	GINI
Poland	—	—	—	—	—	x
Portugal	x	x	x	x	x	—
Republic of Korea	x	x	x	x	x	x
Romania	—	—	—	—	—	—
Rwanda	x	x	x	x	x	—
Saudi Arabia	—	x	—	x	x	—
Senegal	x	x	x	x	x	x
Sierra Leone	x	x	x	x	x	x
Singapore	x	—	x	x	—	—
Somalia	x	x	x	x	x	—
Spain	x	x	x	x	x	x
Sri Lanka	x	—	x	x	x	x
Sudan	x	x	x	x	x	—
Sweden	x	x	x	x	x	x
Switzerland	x	x	x	x	x	x
Syria	x	x	x	x	x	—
Tanzania	x	x	x	x	x	x
Thailand	x	x	x	x	x	x
Togo	x	x	x	x	x	—
Trinidad-Tobago	x	—	x	x	—	x
Tunisia	x	x	x	x	x	x
Turkey	x	x	x	x	x	x
Uganda	x	—	x	x	—	—
United Kingdom	x	x	x	x	x	x
Upper Volta	x	x	x	x	x	—
Uruguay	—	x	—	x	x	x
United States	x	x	x	x	x	x
USSR	x	—	x	—	—	—
Venezuela	x	x	x	x	x	x
Vietnam	x	x	x	x	x	—
Yugoslavia	x	x	x	x	x	x
Zaire	x	x	x	x	x	—
Zambia	x	x	x	x	x	x
Zimbabwe	—	—	—	x	—	x

[a]An x indicates that data are available for the variables in column heads listed above plus all of the dependent variables, foreign and sectoral investment, women's share of tertiary education in 1970, and kilowatt hours per capita. For variable definitions, see Table 4.1.

Appendix B

COUNTRIES USED IN ANALYSES OF FERTILITY BEHAVIOR

Country	TRSTR	CMCON	GINI	INFMORT	FAMPLAN
Afghanistan	—	x[a]	—	x	x
Albania	—	—	—·	—	—
Algeria	x	x	—	x	x
Angola	—	—	—	x	x
Argentina	x	x	x	—	x
Australia	x	x	x	x	—
Austria	x	x	x	x	—
Belgium	x	x	—	x	—
Benin	x	x	x	x	x
Bolivia	—	x	x	x	x
Brazil	x	x	x	x	x
Bulgaria	—	—	x	x	—
Burma	x	x	x	x	x
Burundi	—	—	—	x	x
Central African Republic	x	—	—	x	x
Cambodia	x	x	—	x	x
Cameroon	x	—	—	x	x
Canada	x	—	x	x	—
Chile	x	x	x	x	x
Colombia	x	x	x	x	x
Costa Rica	x	x	x	x	x
Czechoslovakia	x	x	x	x	—
Denmark	x	x	x	x	—
Dominican Republic	—	x	—	x	x
Ecuador	—	x	x	x	x
El Salvador	x	x	x	x	x
Ethiopia	x	x	—	x	x
Egypt	x	x	x	x	x
Finland	x	x	x	x	—
France	x	x	x	x	—
German Democratic Republic	—	—	x	x	—
German Federal Republic	x	x	x	x	—

(continued)

159

Bibliography

Allman, J. (ed.). 1978. Women's Status and Fertility in the Muslim World. New York: Praeger.

Arizpe, L. 1977. "Women in the Informal Labor Sector: The Case of Mexico City." Signs 3(1):25-37.

Awoskika, K. 1976. "Nigerian Women in Distributive Trade." Paper presented at Conference on Women and Development, Wellesley College.

Ballmer-Cao, T., J. Scheiddegger, V. Bornschier, and P. Heintz. 1979. Compendium of Data for World-System Analyses. Zurich: Soziologisches Institut der Universität Zurich.

Bhattacharyya, A. 1975. "Income Inequality and Fertility: A Comparative View." Population Studies 29(1):5-19.

Birdsall, N. 1977. "Analytical Approaches to the Relationship of Population Growth and Development." Population and Development Review 3:63-102.

____. 1976. "Women and Population Studies: Review Essay." Signs 1(3):699-712.

Blake, J. 1974. "The Changing Status of Women in Developed Countries." Scientific American 231 (Dec.):137-47.

____ and P. Das Guptas. 1977. "Reproductive Motivation Versus Contraceptive Technology: Is Recent American Experience an Exception?" Population and Development Review 1:193-253.

Blumberg, R. 1979. "A Paradigm for Predicting the Position of Women." In Sex Roles and Social Policy, edited by J. Lipman-Blumen and J. Bernard. Beverly Hills, Calif.: Sage, pp. 113-42.

____. 1978. Stratification: Socioeconomic and Sexual Inequality. Dubuque, Ia.: William Brown.

____. 1976. "Fairy Tales and Facts: Economy, Family, Fertility, and the Female." In Women and World Development, edited by I. Tinker and M. Bramsen. Washington, D.C.: Overseas Development Council, pp. 12-22.

Bollen, K., and S. Ward. 1980. "Ratio Variables in Aggregate Data Analysis." In Aggregate Data Analysis, edited by E. Borgatta and D. Jackson. Beverly Hills, Calif.: Sage, pp. 60-79.

Bornschier, V. 1978. Multinational Corporations in the World Economy and National Development. Bulletin 32. Zurich: Soziologisches Institut der Universität Zurich.

____ and T. Ballmer-Cao. 1979. "Income Inequality: A Cross-National Study." American Sociological Review 44:487-506.

____ and C. Chase-Dunn. In press. Transnational Corporations and Underdevelopment. New York: Praeger.

____, ____, and R. Rubinson. 1978. "Cross-national Evidence of the Effects of Foreign Investment and Aid on Economic Growth and Inequality: A Survey of the Findings and A Re-analysis." American Journal of Sociology 84:651-83.

Bose, A. 1979. "Some Methodological Issues on Women's Work." In Women and Development in Southeast Asia, edited by R. Jahan and H. Papanek. Dacca: Bangladesh Institute of Law and International Affairs, pp. 117-27.

Boserup, E. 1970. Woman's Role in Economic Development. New York: St. Martin's Press.

Bossen, L. 1984. The Redivision of Labor. Albany: State University of New York Press.

____. 1975. "Women in Modernizing Societies." American Ethnologist 2:587-601.

Boulding, E. 1977. Women in the Twentieth Century World. New York: Halstead Press.

____, S. Nuss, D. Carson, and M. Greenstein. 1976. Handbook of International Data on Women. New York: Halstead Press.

Braverman, H. 1974. Labor and Monopoly Capital. New York: Monthly Review.

Bruce, J. 1976. "Women's Organizations: A Resource for Family Planning and Development." Family Planning Perspectives 8 (Nov.-Dec.):291-97.

Bureau of Labor Statistics. 1980. Perspectives on Working Women: A Databook. Bulletin 2080. Washington, D.C.: U.S. Government Printing Office.

Buvinic, M., and N. Youssef, with B. Von Elm. 1978. Women-Headed Households: The Ignored Factor in Development Planning. Washington, D.C.: International Center for Research on Women.

Caldwell, J. 1982. Theory of Fertility Decline. New York: Academic Press.

____. 1976. "Toward a Restatement of Demographic Transition Theory." Population and Development Review 3:321-66.

Cardoso, F., and E. Faletto. 1979. Dependency and Development in Latin America, translated by M. Urquidi. Berkeley: University of California Press.

Carr, M. 1978. Appropriate Technology for African Women. New York: United Nations.

Chaney, E. 1979. Supermadre: Women in Politics in Latin America. Latin American Monographs No. 50. Austin: University of Texas Press.

____. 1975. "The Mobilization of Women: Three Societies." In Women Cross-Culturally: Challenge and Change, edited by R. Rohrlich-Leavitt. The Hague: Mouton, pp. 472-89.

____. 1973. "Women and Population: Some Key Policy, Research and Action Issues." In Population and Politics: New Directions for Political Scientists, edited by R. Clinton. Lexington, Mass.: Lexington Books, pp. 233-46.

____ and M. Schmink. 1980. "Women and Modernization: Access to Tools." In Sex and Class in Latin America, edited by J. Nash and H. Safa. New York: Bergin, pp. 160-82.

Chase-Dunn, C. 1975. "Dependence, Development and Inequality." American Sociological Review 40:720-38.

_____ and R. Rubinson. 1979. "Cycles, Trends, and New Departures in World-System Development." In National Development and the World System, edited by J. Meyer and M. Hannan. Chicago: University of Chicago Press, pp. 279-96.

Chaudhury, R. 1979. "Female Status and Fertility Behavior in a Metropolitan Urban Area of Bangladesh." In Women and Development in Southeast Asia, edited by R. Jahan and H. Papanek. Dacca: Bangladesh Institute of Law and International Affairs, pp. 319-51.

Chinchilla, N. 1977. "Industrialization, Monopoly Capital, and Women's Work in Guatemala." Signs 3(1):38-56.

Cho, U., and P. Koo. 1983. Capital Accumulation, Women's Work, and Informal Economies in Korea. Working Papers on Women in International Development No. 21. East Lansing: Michigan State University, Office of Women in International Development.

Chodorow, N. 1979. "Mothering, Male Dominance, and Capitalism." In Capitalist Patriarchy and the Case for Socialist Feminism, edited by Z. Eisenstein. New York: Monthly Review Press, pp. 83-106.

Coale, A. 1973. "The Demographic Transition Reconsidered." In International Population Conference, Vol. I. Liege, Belgium: International Union for Scientific Study of Population, p. 65.

Collver, A., and E. Langlois. 1962. "The Female Labor Force in Metropolitan Areas: An International Comparison." Economic Development and Cultural Change 10:367-85.

Concepcion, M. 1974. "Female Labor Force Participation and Fertility." International Labor Review 109(5/6):503-18.

Coser, R. L. 1981. "Where Have All the Women Gone? Like Sediment of a Good Wine, They Have Sunk to the Bottom." In Access to Power: Cross-national Studies of Women and Elites, edited by C. Epstein and R. L. Coser. London: George Allen & Unwin, pp. 16-36.

Cramer, J. 1980. "Fertility and Female Employment." American Sociological Review 45:167-90.

Davidson, M. 1977. "Female Work Status and Fertility in Latin America." In The Fertility of Working Women, edited by S. Kupinsky. New York: Praeger, pp. 342-54.

Davis, K., and S. Blake. 1956. "Social Structure and Fertility: An Analytical Framework." Economic Development and Cultural Change 4:211-35.

Deere, C. 1976. "Rural Women's Subsistence Production in the Capitalist Peripheries." The Review of Radical Political Economics 8(1):9-17.

____, J. Humphries, and M. Leon de Leal. 1982. "Class and Historical Analysis for the Study of Women and Economic Change." In Women's Roles and Population Trends in the Third World, edited by R. Anker, M. Buvinic, and N. Youssef. London: International Labor Office, pp. 87-116.

____ and M. Leon de Leal. 1981. "Peasant Production, Proletarianization, and the Sexual Division of Labor in the Andes." Signs 7(2):338-60.

Delacroix, J. 1978. "Modernizing Institutions, Mobilization, and Third World Development: A Cross-National Study." American Journal of Sociology 84(1):123-50.

____ and C. Ragin. 1981. "Economic Dependency, State Efficacy, and Peripheral Countries." American Journal of Sociology 86(6):1311-47.

Demeny, P. 1979. "On the End of the Population Explosion." Population and Development Review 5(1):141-62.

Dixon, R. 1982. "Women in Agriculture: Counting the Labor Force in Developing Countries." Population and Development Review 8(3):539-66.

____. 1978a. "On Drawing Policy Conclusions From Multiple Regressions: Some Queries and Dilemmas." Studies in Family Planning 9(10-11):286-287.

____. 1978b. Rural Women at Work. Baltimore: John Hopkins University Press.

____. 1975. Women's Rights and Fertility. Reports on Popula-
tion Family Planning No. 17. New York: Population Council.

Durand, J. 1975. The Labor Force in Economic Development.
Princeton, N.J.: Princeton University Press.

Ehrenreich, B., and A. Fuentes. 1981. "Life on the Global
Assembly Line." Ms. 9(7):52-59, 71.

Eisenstein, Z. 1982. "The Sexual Politics of the New Right:
Understanding the 'Crisis of Liberalism' for the 1980s."
Signs 7(3):567-88.

____. 1979. "Developing a Theory of Capitalist Patriarchy and
Socialist Feminism." In Capitalist Patriarchy and the Case
for Socialist Feminism, edited by Z. Eisenstein. New York:
Monthly Review Press, pp. 5-40.

El Saadawi, N. 1980. The Hidden Face of Eve. London: George
Allen & Unwin.

Elson, D., and R. Pearson. 1981a. "'Nimble fingers make cheap
workers': An Analysis of Women's Employment in Third World
Export Manufacturing." Feminist Review (Spring):87-107.

____ and ____. 1981b. "The Subordination of Women and the
Internationalisation of Factory Production." In Of Marriage
and the Market: Women's Subordination in International
Perspective, edited by K. Young, C. Wolkowitz, and
R. McCullagh. London: CSE, pp. 144-66.

Elu de Lenero, C. 1980. "Women's Work and Fertility." In
Sex and Class in Latin America, edited by J. Nash and
H. Safá. New York: Bergin, pp. 46-68.

Epstein, C. 1981a. "Women and Elites: A Cross-national
Perspective." In Access to Power: Cross-national Studies
of Women and Elites, edited by C. Epstein and R. L. Coser.
London: George Allen & Unwin, pp. 3-15.

____. 1981b. "Women and Power: The Roles of Women in Politics
in the United States." In Access to Power: Cross-national
Studies of Women and Elites, edited by C. Epstein and R. L.
Coser. London: George Allen & Unwin, pp. 124-46.

Evans, P. 1979. Dependent Development. Princeton, N.J.: Princeton University Press.

____ and M. Timberlake, 1980. "Dependence, Inequality and Growth in Less Developed Countries." American Sociological Review 45(4):531-52.

Fernández-Kelly, M. 1983. For We Are Sold: I and My People: Women and Industry in Mexico's Frontier. Albany: State University of New York Press.

____. 1980. "The 'Maquila' Women." NACLA Report on the Americas 14(5):14-19.

Fiala, R. 1983. "Inequality and the Service Sector in Less Developed Countries." American Sociological Review 48:421-27.

Flexner, E. 1975. Century of Struggle. Cambridge, Mass.: Harvard University Press.

Flynn, P. 1980. "Women Challenge the Myth." NACLA Report on the Americas 14:20-35.

Fong, M. 1975. Female Labor Force Participation in A Modernizing Society: Malaya and Singapore, 1921-1957. Papers of the East-West Population Institute No. 34. Honolulu: East-West Center.

____. 1973. "Female Labor Force Participation and Fertility: Some Methodological Considerations." Social Biology 23(1):45-54.

Frank, A. 1966. "The Development of Underdevelopment." Monthly Review 18:17-31.

Freeman, J. 1975. The Politics of Women's Liberation. Palo Alto, Calif.: Mayfield.

Friedl, E. 1975. Women and Men: An Anthropologist's View. New York: Holt, Rinehart & Winston.

Friedlander, S., and M. Silver. 1967. "A Quantitative Study of the Determinants of Fertility Behavior." Demography 4:30-61.

Froebel, F., J. Heinrichs, and O. Kreye. 1980. The New International Division of Labour. Cambridge: Cambridge University Press.

Galtung, J. 1971. "A Structural Theory of Imperialism." Journal of Peace Research 2:89-117.

Germain, A. 1975. "Status and Roles of Women as Factors in Fertility Behavior: A Policy Analysis." Studies in Family Planning 6(7):192-200.

Gordon, L. 1977. Woman's Body, Woman's Right. New York: Schocken.

Grossman, R. 1978/79. "Women's Place in the Integrated Circuit." Southeast Asia Chronicle 66: Pacific Research 9:2-17.

Hafkin, N., and E. Bay (eds.). 1976. Women in Africa: Studies in Social and Economic Change. Stanford, Calif.: Stanford University Press.

Hartmann, H. 1976. "Capitalism, Patriarchy, and Job Segregation by Sex." In Women in the Workplace, edited by M. Blaxall and B. Reagan. Chicago: University of Chicago Press, pp. 137-170.

Hass, P. 1972. "Maternal Role Incompatibility and Fertility in Urban Latin America." Journal of Social Issues 28:111-128.

Hawley, A. 1950. Human Ecology. New York: Ronalds Press.

Henry, F., and P. Wilson. 1975. "The Status of Women in Caribbean Societies: An Overview of Their Social, Economic, and Sexual Roles." Social and Economic Studies 24(2):165-98.

Hernandez, D. 1981. "A Note on Measuring the Independent Impact of Family Planning Programs on Fertility Declines." Demography 18(4):627-34.

Hohm, C. 1975. "Social Security and Fertility: An International Perspective." Demography 12(4):629-44.

Hosken, F. 1977. International Directory of Women's Development Organizations. Washington, D.C.: Agency for International Development.

Hout, M. 1981. "The Role of Household Production and Commodity Trade in Latin American Fertility: 1915-1975." Unpublished paper, University of Arizona.

____. 1980. "Trade Dependence and Fertility in Hispanic America." In Studies of the Modern World-System, edited by A. Bergesen. New York: Academic Press, pp. 159-88.

Huber, J. 1980. "Will U.S. Fertility Decline Toward Zero?" The Sociological Quarterly 21:481-92.

Hull, V. 1977. "Fertility, Women's Work, and Economic Class: A Case Study from Southeast Asia." In The Fertility of Working Women, edited by S. Kupinsky. New York: Praeger, pp. 35-80.

Huntington, S. 1975. "Issues in Woman's Role in Economic Development." Journal of Marriage and the Family 37(4): 1001-13.

Hurwitz, E. 1977. "The International Sisterhood of Women." In Becoming Visible: Women in European History, edited by R. Bridenthal and E. Koonz. Boston: Houghton Mifflin, pp. 325-45.

Inkeles, A., and D. Smith. 1975. Becoming Modern. Cambridge, Mass.: Harvard University Press.

International Center for Research on Women. 1980a. The Productivity of Women in Developing Countries: Measurement Issues and Recommendations. AID/otr/C-1801. Washington, D.C.: Agency for International Development.

____. 1980b. Keeping Women Out: A Structural Analysis of Women's Employment in Developing Countries. Washington, D.C.: Agency for International Development.

International Labor Office. 1979. The Cost of Social Security. Ninth International Inquiry, 1972-74. Geneva: International Labor Office.

_____. 1977. Labor Force Estimates and Projections, 1950-2000. Geneva: International Labor Office.

Jackman, R. 1980. "A Note on the Measurement of Growth Ratios in Crossnational Research." American Journal of Sociology 86:604-17.

Jacquette, J. 1980. "Female Political Participation in Latin America." In Sex and Class in Latin America, edited by J. Nash and H. Safa. New York: Bergin, pp. 211-44.

Jaffe, A., and K. Azumi. 1960. "The Birthrate and Cottage Industries in Underdeveloped Countries." Economic Development and Cultural Change 9(1):52-63.

Jahan, R. 1979a. "Introduction." In Women and Development in Southeast Asia, edited by R. Jahan and H. Papanek. Dacca: Bangladesh Institute of Law and International Affairs, pp. 1-20.

_____. 1979b. "Public Policies, Women and Development: Reflections on a Few Structural Problems." In Women and Development in Southeast Asia, edited by R. Jahan and H. Papanek. Dacca: Bangladesh Institute of Law and International Affairs, pp. 55-70.

_____ and H. Papanek. 1979. Women and Development in Southeast Asia. Dacca: Bangladesh Institute of Law and International Affairs.

Jain, D., N. Singh, and M. Chand. 1979. "Women's Work: Methodological Issues." In Women and Development in Southeast Asia, edited by R. Jahan and H. Papanek. Dacca: Bangladesh Institute of Law and International Affairs, pp. 128-70.

Jain, S. 1975. Size Distribution of Income: A Compilation of Data. Washington, D.C.: World Bank.

Jelin, E. 1980. "The Bahiana in the Labor Force in Slavador, Brazil." In Sex and Class in Latin America, edited by J. Nash and H. Safa. New York: Bergin, pp. 129-46.

_____. 1977. "Migration and Labor Force Participation of Latin American Women: The Domestic Servants in the Cities." Signs 3(1):129-41.

Joseph, G. 1980. "Caribbean Women: The Impact of Race, Sex, and Class." In Comparative Perspectives of Third World Women, edited by B. Lindsay. New York: Praeger, pp. 143-61.

Jules-Rosette, B. 1982. Women's Work in the Informal Sector: A Zambian Case Study. Working Papers on Women in International Development No. 3. East Lansing: Michigan State University, Office of Women in International Development.

Kamerman, S. 1979. "Work and Family in Industrialized Societies." Signs 4(4):632-50.

_____ and A. Kahn (eds.). 1978. Family Policy: Government and Families in Fourteen Countries. New York: Columbia University Press.

Kasarda, J. D. 1971. "Economic Structure and Fertility: A Comparative Analysis." Demography 8(3):307-17.

Kelly, W., P. Cutright, and D. Hittle. 1976. "Comment on Charles Hohm's 'Social Security and Fertility.'" Demography 13(4):581-86.

Kentor, J. 1981. "Structural Determinants of Peripheral Urbanization." American Sociological Review 46:201-11.

Knodel, J. 1977. "Family Limitation and the Fertility Transition: Evidence from the Age Patterns of Fertility in Europe and Asia." Population Studies 31:219-49.

Koo, H., and P. Smith. 1983. "Migration, the Urban Informal Sector, and Earnings in the Philippines." The Sociological Quarterly 24(2):219-32.

Kupinsky, S. 1977a. "The Fertility of Working Women in the United States: Historical Trends and Theoretical Perspectives." In The Fertility of Working Women, edited by S. Kupinsky. New York: Praeger, pp. 188-249.

_____. 1977b. "Overview and Policy Implications." In The Fertility of Working Women, edited by S. Kupinsky. New York: Praeger, pp. 369-80.

_____. 1971. "Nonfamilial Activity and Socio-Economic Differentials in Fertility." Demography 8(3):353-68.

Lapidus, G. 1978. _Women in Soviet Society: Equality, Development, and Social Change._ Berkeley: University of California Press.

Leghorn, L., and K. Parker. 1981. _Women's Worth: Sexual Economics and The World of Women._ Boston: Routledge & Kegan Paul.

Leis, N. 1974. "Women in Groups, Ijaw Women's Associations." In _Woman, Culture and Society,_ edited by N. Hafkin and E. Bay. Stanford, Calif.: Stanford University Press, pp. 223-42.

Lewis, B. 1976. "The Limitations of Group Action Among Entrepreneurs: The Market Women of Abidjaw, Ivory Coast." In _Women in Africa,_ edited by N. Hafkin and E. Bay. Stanford, Calif.: Stanford University Press, pp. 136-56.

Lewis, S. 1980. "African Women and National Development." In _Comparative Perspectives on Third World Women,_ edited by B. Lindsay. New York: Praeger, pp. 31-54.

Lim, L. 1983a. "Are Multinationals the Problem? A Debate." _Multinational Monitor_ 4(8):12-16.

_____. 1983b. "Capitalism, Imperialism, and Patriarchy." In _Women, Men, and the International Division of Labor,_ edited by J. Nash and M. Fernández-Kelly. Albany: State University of New York Press, pp. 70-92.

_____. 1978. _Workers in Multinational Corporations: The Case of the Electronics Industry in Malaysia and Singapore._ Michigan Occasional Papers in Women's Studies No. 9. Ann Arbor: University of Michigan.

Lindsay, B. (ed.). 1980. _Comparative Perspectives of Third World Women._ New York: Praeger.

Little, K. 1973. _African Women in Towns: An Aspect of Africa's Social Revolution._ Cambridge: Cambridge University Press.

Long, S. 1979. "The Continuing Debate Over the Use of Ratio Variables: Facts and Fiction." In _Sociological Methodology 1980,_ edited by K. Schuessler. San Francisco: Jossey-Bass, pp. 37-67.

Lunday, J., and M. Timberlake. In press. "Labor Force Structure in the Zones of the World-Economy: 1950-70." In Urbanization in the World-Economy, edited by M. Timberlake. New York: Academic Press.

McBride, T. 1977. "The Long Road Home: Women's Work and Industrialization." In Becoming Visible: Women in European History, edited by R. Bridenthal and E. Koonz. Boston: Houghton Mifflin, pp. 280-95.

McGrath, P. 1976. The Unfinished Assignment: Equal Education for Women. Worldwatch Paper No. 7. New York: Worldwatch Institute.

Mass, B. 1976. Population Target. Brampton, Ontario: Chartus.

Matyepse, I. 1977. "Underdevelopment and African Women." Journal of Southern African Affairs 21:6.

Mauldin, W., and B. Berelson. 1978. "Conditions of Fertility Decline in Developing Countries, 1965-75." Studies in Family Planning 9(5):89-147.

Mazumdar, V. 1979. "Women, Development and Public Policy." In Women and Development in Southeast Asia, edited by R. Jahan and H. Papanek. Dacca: Bangladesh Institute of Law and International Affairs, pp. 39-54.

Meillassoux, C. 1981. Maidens, Meal and Money. Cambridge: Cambridge University Press.

Mernissi, F. 1977. Beyond the Veil: Male-Female Dynamics in a Modern Muslim World. New York: Halstead Press.

Meyer, J., M. Hannan, R. Rubinson, and G. Thomas. 1979. "National Economic Development, 1950-70: Social and Political Factors." In National Development and The World System, edited by J. Meyer and M. Hannan. Chicago: University of Chicago Press, pp. 85-116.

Milkman, R. 1976. "Women's Work and the Economic Crisis: Some Lessons from the Great Depression." The Review of Radical Political Economics 8(1):73-97.

175

Mintz, S. 1971. "Men, Women and Trade." Comparative Studies in Society and History 13:247-69.

Miranda, G. 1977. "Women's Labor Force Participation in a Developing Society: The Case of Brazil." Signs 3(1):261-74.

Mueller, E. 1976. "The Economic Value of Children in Peasant Agriculture." In Population and Development, edited by R. Ridker. Baltimore: Johns Hopkins University Press, pp. 98-153.

Mueller, L. 1977. "Women and Men, Power and Powerlessness in Lesotho." Signs 3(1):154-66.

Müller, R. 1979. "The Multinational Corporation and the Underdevelopment of the Third World." In The Political Economy of Development and Underdevelopment (second edition), edited by C. Wilber. New York: Random House, pp. 151-78.

Mullings, L. 1976. "Women and Economic Change in Africa." In Women in Africa, edited by N. Hafkin and E. Bay. Stanford, Calif.: Stanford University Press, pp. 239-64.

Nader, L., and J. Collier. 1978. "Justice—A Woman Blindfolded?" In Women in the Courts, edited by W. Hepperle and L. Crites. Williamsburg, Va.: National Center for State Courts, pp. 202-221.

Nash, J. 1983. "The Impact of the Changing International Division of Labor on Different Sectors of the Labor Force." In Women, Men and the International Division of Labor, edited by J. Nash and M. Fernández-Kelly. Albany: State University of New York Press, pp. 3-38.

_____. 1980. "A Critique of Social Science Roles in Latin America." In Sex and Class in Latin America, edited by J. Nash and H. Safa. New York: Bergin, pp. 1-21.

_____ and M. Fernández-Kelly (eds.). 1983. Women, Men, and the International Division of Labor. Albany: State University of New York Press.

Neumann, A. L. 1978/79. "'Hospitality Girls' in the Philippines." Southeast Asia Chronicle 66/Pacific Research 9:18-22.

Newland, K. 1980. Women, Men, and The Division of Labor. Worldwatch Paper No. 37. Washington, D.C.: Worldwatch Institute.

____. 1979. The Sisterhood of Man. New York: Norton.

____. 1977. Women and Population Growth: Choice Beyond Childbearing. Worldwatch Paper No. 16. New York: Worldwatch Institute.

North American Congress On Latin America [NACLA]. 1977. "Electronics: The Global Industry." NACLA Report 9(4).

Nuss, S., and Majka, L. 1983. "The Economic Integration of Women: A Cross-national Investigation." Work and Occupations 10:29-48.

Okonjo, K. 1979. "Rural Women's Credit Systems: A Nigerian Example." Studies in Family Planning 10(11/12):326-31.

Oppenheimer, V. 1970. The Female Labor Force in the United States. Population Monograph No. 5. Berkeley: University of California Press.

Papanek, H. 1979a. "Introduction." In Women and Development in Southeast Asia, edited by R. Jahan and H. Papanek. Dacca: Bangladesh Institute of Law and International Affairs, pp. 23-36.

____. 1979b. "Development Planning for Women: The Implications of Women's Work." In Women and Development in Southeast Asia, edited by R. Jahan and H. Papanek. Dacca: Bangladesh Institute of Law and International Affairs, pp. 170-201.

____. 1978. "Comment on Gusfield's Review Essay on Becoming Modern." American Journal of Sociology 83:157-11.

____. 1976. "Women in Cities: Problems and Perspectives." In Women and World Development, edited by I. Tinker and M. Bramsen. Washington, D.C.: Overseas Development Council, pp. 54-69.

____. 1971. "Purdah in Pakistan: Seclusion and Modern Occupations for Women." Journal of Marriage and the Family 33(3):517-30.

Paukert, F. 1973. "Income Distribution at Different Levels of Development: A Survey of Evidence." International Labor Review 108:97-125.

Piepmeier, K., and T. Adkins. 1973. "The Status of Women and Fertility." Journal of Biosocial Science 5:507-20.

Portes, A. In press. "The Informal Sector and the World-Economy: Notes on the Structure of Subsidized Labor." In Urbanization and the World-System, edited by M. Timberlake. New York: Academic Press.

____. 1976. "On the Sociology of National Development: Theories and Issues." American Journal of Sociology 32: 55-85.

____ and J. Walton. 1981. Labor, Class, and the International System. New York: Academic Press.

Rainwater, L. 1965. Family Design: Marital Sexuality, Family Size, and Contraception. Chicago: Aldine.

Ramirez, F. 1981. "Statism, Equality, and Housewifery: A Cross-National Analysis." Pacific Sociological Review 24(2): 175-195.

____. 1980. "World Political Economy and Female Participation in Higher Education." Paper presented at American Sociological Association meetings, New York.

____ and G. Thomas. 1981. "Structural Antecedents and the Consequences of Statism." In Dynamics of World Development, edited by R. Rubinson. Beverly Hills, Calif.: Sage, pp. 139-66.

____ and J. Weiss. 1979. "The Political Incorporation of Women." In National Development and the World System, edited by J. Meyer and M. Hannan. Chicago: University of Chicago Press, pp. 238-49.

Repetto, R. 1979. Economic Equality and Fertility in Developing Countries. Baltimore: Johns Hopkins University Press.

____. 1974. "The Relationship of the Size Distribution of Income to Fertility and the Implications for Development Policy." In

Population Policies and Economic Development, edited by
T. King. Baltimore: Johns Hopkins University Press,
pp. 149-66.

Robert, A. 1983. "The Effects of the International Division of
Labor on Female Workers in the Textile and Clothing Industries." Development and Change 14:19-37.

Robertson, C. 1976. "Ga Women and Socioeconomic Change in
Accra, Ghana." In Women in Africa, edited by N. Hatkin
and E. Bay. Stanford, Calif.: Stanford University Press,
pp. 111-34.

Rogers, S. 1978. "Women's Place: A Critical Review of
Anthropological Theory." Comparative Studies in Society
and History 20(1):123-62.

Rosaldo, M. 1980. "The Use and Abuse of Anthropology:
Reflections on Feminism and Cross-Cultural Understanding."
Signs 5:389-417.

____. 1974. "Women, Culture, and Society: A Theoretical
Overview." In Women, Culture and Society, edited by
M. Rosaldo and L. Lamphere. Stanford, Calif.: Stanford
University Press, pp. 17-42.

Rosen, B., and A. Simmons. 1971. "Industrialization, Family
and Fertility: Structural-psychological Analysis of the
Brazilian Case." Demography 8(1):49-69.

Rosenberg, T. J. 1982. "Female Industrial Employment and
Protective Labor Legislation in Bogota, Colombia." Journal
of Interamerican Studies and World Affairs 24(1):59-80.

Rubin, G. 1975. "The Traffic in Women: Notes on the 'Political
Economy of Sex.'" In Toward An Anthropology of Women,
edited by R. Reiter. New York: Monthly Review Press,
pp. 157-210.

Rubinson, R. 1976. "The World-Economy and Distribution of
Income." American Sociological Review 41:638-59.

Sadik, N. 1974. "A Stronger Voice for Women." Equilibrium
11(11):34-35.

Safa, H. 1981. "Runaway Shops and Female Employment: The Search for Cheap Labor." Signs 7(2):418-33.

____. 1977. "The Changing Class Composition of the Female Labor Force in Latin America." Latin American Perspectives 4(Fall):126-36.

Saffioti, H. 1978. Women in Class Society. New York: Monthly Review Press.

____. 1977. "Women, Mode of Production, and Social Formations." Latin American Perspectives 4 (Winter/Spring):27-37.

____. 1975. "Female Labor and Capitalism in the United States and Brazil." In Women Cross-Culturally: Challenge and Change, edited by R. Rohrlich-Leavitt. The Hague: Mouton, pp. 59-94.

Safilios-Rothschild, C. 1982. "Female Power, Autonomy, and Demographic Change in the Third World." In Women's Roles and Population Trends in the Third World, edited by R. Anker, M. Buvinic, and N. Youssef. London: International Labor Office, pp. 117-32.

____. 1977. "The Relationship Between Women's Work and Fertility: Some Methodological and Theoretical Issues." In The Fertility of Working Women, edited by S. Kupinsky. New York: Praeger, pp. 355-68.

Salaff, J. 1981. Working Daughters of Hong Kong. Cambridge: Cambridge University Press.

Sanday, P. 1981. Female Power and Male Dominance. Cambridge: Cambridge University Press.

____. 1974. "Female Status in the Public Domain." In Woman, Culture and Society, edited by M. Rosaldo and L. Lamphere. Stanford, Calif.: Stanford University Press, pp. 189-206.

Sanzone, D. 1981. "Women in Politics: A Study of Political Leadership in the United Kingdom, France, and the Federal Republic of Germany." In Access to Power: Cross-National Studies of Women and Elites, edited by C. Epstein and R. L. Coser. London: George Allen & Unwin, pp. 37-52.

Scanzoni, J., and M. McMurry. 1972. "Continuities in the Explanation of Fertility Control." Journal of Marriage and the Family 34:315-21.

Schmink, M. 1977. "Dependent Development and the Division of Labor by Sex: Venezuela." Latin American Perspectives 4(1/2):153-79.

Scrimshaw, S. 1978. "Infant Mortality and Behavior in the Regulation of Family Size." Population and Development Review 4(3):383-403.

Seidman, A. 1981. "Women and the Development of Under-development: The African Experience." In Women and Technological Change in Developing Countries, edited by R. Dauber and M. Lain. NAAS Selected Symposium No. 53. Boulder, Colo.: Westview, pp. 109-26.

Semyonov, M. 1980. "The Social Context of Women's Labor Force Participation: A Comparative Analysis." American Journal of Sociology 86:534-50.

Shapiro, H. 1980. "The Many Realities." NACLA Report on the Americas 14(5):2-13.

Shyrock, H., J. Siegel, and E. Stockwell. 1976. The Methods and Materials of Demography. New York: Academic Press.

Siegel, L. 1978/79. "Orchestrating Dependency." Southeast Asia Chronicle 66; Pacific Research 9:24-27.

Simms, R., and E. Dumor. 1976/77. "Women in the Urban Economy of Ghana: Associational Activity and the Enclave Economy." African Urban Notes 2(3):43-64.

Simon, J. 1977. The Economics of Population Growth, Princeton, N.J.: Princeton University Press.

____. 1976. "Income, Wealth, and Their Distribution as Policy Tools in Fertility Control." In Population and Development, edited by R. Ridker. Baltimore: Johns Hopkins University Press, pp. 36-76.

Skocpol, T. 1976. "Wallerstein's World Capitalist System: A Theoretical and Historical Critique." American Journal of Sociology 82:1075-90.

181

Sokoloff, N. 1980. Between Money and Love. New York: Praeger.

Standing, G. 1978. Labor Force Participation and Development. Geneva: International Labor Office.

Stolte-Heiskanen, V. 1977. "Fertility and Women's Employment Outside the Home in Western Europe." In The Fertility of Working Women, edited by S. Kupinsky. New York: Praeger, pp. 250-80.

Stycos, J., and R. Weller. 1967. "Female Working Roles and Fertility." Demography 4(1):210-17.

Sudarkasa, N. 1977. "Women and Migration in Contemporary West Africa." Signs 3(1):178-89.

Szabady, E. 1977. "Fertility and Women's Employment in the Socialist Countries of Eastern Europe." In The Fertility of Working Women, edited by S. Kupinsky. New York: Praeger, pp. 281-316.

Tangri, S. 1976. "A Feminist Perspective on Some Ethical Issues in Population Programs." Signs 1(4):895-904.

Teitelbaum, M. 1975. "Relevance of Demographic Transition Theory for Developing Countries." Science 188:420-25.

Tilly, C. 1978. Historical Studies of Changing Fertility. Princeton, N.J.: Princeton University Press.

Timberlake, M. In press. Urbanization and the World-System. New York: Academic Press.

_____ and J. Kentor. 1983. "Economic Dependence, Overurbanization, and Economic Growth: A Study of Less Developed Countries." The Sociological Quarterly 24(4):489-508.

Tinker, I., and M. Bramsen. 1976. "The Adverse Impact of Development on Women." In Women and World Development, edited by I. Tinker and M. B. Bramsen. Washington, D.C.: Overseas Development Council, pp. 22-34.

Todaro, M. 1981. Economic Development in the Third World (second edition). New York: Longman.

Tsui, A., and D. Bogue. 1978. "Declining World Fertility: Trends, Causes and Implications." Population Bulletin 33(4).

Ul Haq, M. 1979. "The Inequities of the Old Economic Order." In The Political Economy of Development and Underdevelopment, edited by C. Wilber. New York: Random House, pp. 179-88.

UNESCO. 1978. Statistical Yearbook. New York: United Nations.

____. 1976. Statistical Yearbook. New York: United Nations.

____. 1972. Statistical Yearbook. New York: United Nations.

United Nations. 1980. "Review and Evaluation of Progress Achieved in the Implementation of the World Plan of Action: Employment." Paper prepared for the World Conference of the United Nations Decade for Women. Copenhagen, Denmark, July 14-30, 1980. A/CONF.94/8.

____. 1976. Demographic Yearbook. New York: United Nations.

____. 1975a. Interregional Seminar on National Machinery to Accelerate the Integration of Women in Development and to Eliminate Discrimination on Grounds of Sex. ST/ESA/SER.B/7. Ottawa, Canada, September 4-17, 1975. New York: United Nations.

____. 1975b. Status of Women and Family Planning. E/CN.6/575/Rev.1. New York: United Nations.

____. 1970. Political Rights of Women. A/8132 and A/81321/Add.1. New York: United Nations.

United Nations Economic Commission for Africa, Human Resources Development Division, African Training and Research Center for Women. 1975. "Women and National Development in African Countries: Some Profound Contradictions." African Studies Review 18(3):47-70.

Van Allen, J. 1976. "African Women, 'Modernization,' and National Liberation." In Women in the World: A Comparative Study, edited by L. Iglitzin and R. Ross. Santa Barbara, Calif.: ABC-Clio, pp. 25-54.

Wachtel, E. 1976. "Minding Her Own Business: Women Shop-
keepers in Nakuru, Kenya." African Urban Notes 2(2):27-
42.

Waite, L. 1982. "U.S. Women at Work." Population Reference
Bureau 36(2).

Wallerstein, I. 1979. The Capitalist World Economy. Cambridge:
Cambridge University Press.

____. 1974. The Modern World System. New York: Academic
Press.

Ward, K. In press. "Women and Urbanization in the World-
System." In Urbanization and the World-System, edited by
M. Timberlake. New York: Academic Press.

____. 1982. "The Influence of the World Economic System on
the Status of Women and Their Fertility Behavior." Ph.D.
Dissertation. Iowa City: University of Iowa.

____ and J. Weiss. 1982. "A Competitive Model of Women's
Labor Force Participation in the United States: 1940-1978.
Paper presented at American Sociological Association meetings,
San Francisco.

Ware, H. 1977. "Women's Work and Fertility in Africa." In
The Fertility of Working Women, edited by S. Kupinsky.
New York: Praeger, pp. 1-34.

Weiss, J. 1978. "A Competitive Model of Women's Labor Force
Participation." Unpublished paper, University of Iowa.

____ and F. Ramirez. 1976. "The Impact of Nation-State
Corporateness on the Status and Participation of Women."
Paper presented at Pacific Sociological Association meetings,
San Diego.

____, ____, and T. Tracy. 1976. "Female Participation in the
Occupational System: A Comparative Institutional Analysis."
Social Problems 23:593-608.

Wellesley Editorial Committee. 1977. "Women and National
Development." Signs 3(1).

184

Wertheimer, B. 1977. We Were There: A History of Working Women in America. New York: Pantheon.

Westoff, C. 1978. "Marriage and Fertility in the Developed Countries." Scientific American 239:51-57.

Whyte, M. K. 1978. The Status of Women in Preindustrial Societies. Princeton, N.J.: Princeton University Press.

Young, I. 1981. "Beyond the Unhappy Marriage: A Critique of the Dual Systems Theory." In Women and Revolution, edited by L. Sargent. Boston: South End Press, pp. 43-70.

Youssef, N. 1982. "The Interrelationship Between the Division of Labor in the Household, Women's Roles, and Their Impact on Fertility." In Women's Roles and Population Trends in The Third World, edited by R. Anker, M. Buvinic, and N. Youssef. London: International Labor Office, pp. 173-201.

____. 1979. "Women's Employment and Fertility: Demographic Transition or Economic Needs of Mothers?" Washington, D.C.: International Center for Research on Women.

____. 1976. "Women in Development: Urban Life and Labor." In Women and World Development, edited by I. Tinker and M. Bramsen. Washington, D.C.: Overseas Development Council, pp. 70-77.

____. 1974. Women and Work in Developing Societies. Berkeley: University of California Press.

____ and S. Hartley. 1979. "Demographic Indicators of The Status of Women in Various Societies." In Sex Roles and Social Policy, edited by J. Lipman-Blumen and J. Bernard. Beverly Hills, Calif.: Sage, pp. 83-112.

method of analysis, 67-68
missing data, 65
model specification, 142-45
modernity theory, 7-8;
    criticism of, 8-9; as in-
    adequate, 9
mortality, see infant mortality

nation(s): core, see core
    nations; developed, see
    developed countries; de-
    veloping, see developing
    countries

organization(s): of women
    workers, 29, see also
    women's organizations
organizational resources:
    fertility and, 50
organizational status: discus-
    sion of, 133
overurbanization, 14

patriarchal ideologies, 18-19
patriarchal mechanisms, 15-19
patriarchal relations: capital-
    ism maintenance and, 16-
    17; definition, 14-15; of
    world-system, 14-15
policy: implications of study
    for, 145-53
political resources: fertility
    and, 50
political status, 34-35; discus-
    sion of, 133
power sharing with experts,
    139-40
production: capitalist commod-
    ity, 10; for export, 11;
    indigenous, restraint of, 10
productive role of women, 15-
    16

ratio variables, 67
raw materials, 10

regression analysis, 114-29
reliability: of data on status
    of women, 143-45
reproductive role of women,
    15-16
research: design, 59-72;
    fertility, 152-53; implica-
    tions of study for, 145-
    53; needed research at
    macro level, 148; needed
    research at micro level,
    148; strategy, 68-72
resources: organizational,
    and fertility, 50; political,
    and fertility, 50; in public
    domain, and status of
    women, 20
revolution: economic, in six-
    teenth century, 10
role: productive, 15-16,
    reproductive, 15-16

sample, 59
service employment, 30-31
service sector: growth of,
    13; women's share of,
    97-98
social differentiation theory,
    7-8; criticism of, 8-9
social setting: as independ-
    ent variable, 65
specification: model, 142-45
state(s): capitalist, becoming
    core nations, 10; discus-
    sion of, 134-35; as inter-
    vening mechanism, 12;
    strength, and economic
    dependency, 13
status of women, 19-39; con-
    trol variables, 82-83;
    correlations on, 110-14;
    data on, 110-14; discus-
    sion of, 131-35; economic,
    see economic status of
    women; educational, and

190

[status of women]
family planning programs, 151; effect on fertility, 107-37; feedback effects of, 146; fertility and, 47, 52-54; as independent variable, 64; organizational, 133; political, 34-35, 133; redefinition of, 21; in regression analysis, 114-18; reliability of data on, 143-45; resources in public domain and, 20; survey of, 21-38; theoretical perspective on, 20-21; validity of data on, 143-45; world-system and, 52-56

technical experts, 14
technology: control over, 11; innovation and, 11
theoretical arguments: summary of, 139-41
theory: dependency, 7-8; of economic development, 7-12; implications of study for, 145-53; linear stages, 7; modernity, see modernity theory; overview, 7-57; social differentiation, see social differentiation theory; women in development, 147; world-system, 8-12
TNC, see transnational corporation
trade dependency, 12; relations, 9-10
trading employment, 26
transnational corporations, 10; employment in developing countries, 27-30, 89, 149; investment by, largest share of, 11
underdevelopment: dependent development and, 11, 25,

39, 49; indirect effects of, 101-03
unionization, 38
urbanization, 42; as intervening mechanism, 12

validity of data on status of women, 143-45
variables: control, 81-82; status-of-women, 82-83; dependency, 76, 81; dependent, 60; independent, 60-64; intervening, 81-82; investment, 76, 81; ratio, 67

women: in development, 147-49; education of, 132-33; legislation for, 35-36; organizations of, 29, 36-37; share of, see women's share; status of, see status of women; workers, organization of, 29
women's organizations, 36-37
women's share: of agricultural sector, 95-97; of economic sectors, 89-92; of industrial sector, 95-97; of labor force, 83-89, 92-97; of service sector, 97-98
world economic system, see world-system
world-system: control of, 10; economic status of women and, 38-43, 140, 145-47; fertility and, 45, 52-54; inequality and, 130-31; nature of, 10; origins of, 10; patriarchal relations of, 14-15; status of women and, 52-54; theory, 8-12

About the Author

KATHRYN B. WARD is an assistant professor of sociology at Southern Illinois University at Carbondale.

Dr. Ward has published and taught in the areas of development, stratification, and gender. Her articles have appeared in Review, Work and Occupations, and several multiauthor volumes on the world-system.

Dr. Ward holds a B.A. from Fort Hays State University, Kansas, and an M.A. and Ph.D. from the University of Iowa, Iowa City.

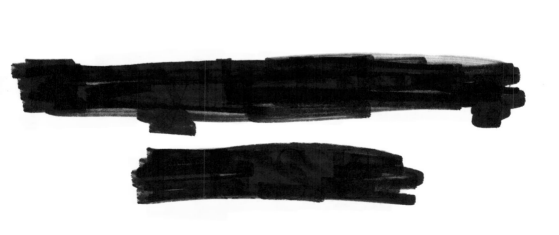